HUMAN ANATOMY AND PHYSIOLOGY

SOFT TISSUE

COMPOSITION, MECHANISMS OF INJURY AND REPAIR

HUMAN ANATOMY AND PHYSIOLOGY

Additional books in this series can be found on Nova's website under the Series tab.

Additional e-books in this series can be found on Nova's website under the e-book tab.

PHYSIOLOGY – LABORATORY AND CLINICAL RESEARCH

Additional books in this series can be found on Nova's website under the Series tab.

Additional e-books in this series can be found on Nova's website under the e-book tab.

HUMAN ANATOMY AND PHYSIOLOGY

SOFT TISSUE

COMPOSITION, MECHANISMS OF INJURY AND REPAIR

ANTONIO J. CHAVEZ RUIZ

AND

JOSE M. ALVAREZ MENDOZA

EDITORS

Nova Science Publishers, Inc.

New York

For permission to use material from this book please contact us:
Telephone 631-231-7269; Fax 631-231-8175
Web Site: http://www.novapublishers.com

NOTICE TO THE READER

Library of Congress Cataloging-in-Publication Data

Library of Congress Control Number: 2012941271

ISBN 978-1-62257-363-9

Published by Nova Science Publishers, Inc. †New York

Contents

Preface

Soft tissue refers to tissues that connect, support, or surround other structures and organs of the body, not being bone. Soft tissue includes tendons, ligaments, fascia, skin, fibrous tissues, fat, and synovial membranes (which are connective tissue), and muscles, nerves and blood vessels (which are not connective tissue). In this book, the authors present current research in the study of the composition, mechanisms of injury and repair of soft tissue. Topics discussed include the soft tissue biomechanics of diabetic foot ulcers; cellular and physiological soft tissue response in hip arthroplasty; peri-implant soft tissues in orthodontic anchorage; connecting tissue injuries and mechanical properties; MRI findings of myopathies in soft tissue; and soft tissue behavior after mandibular symphysis bone graft harvesting.

Chapter I - Diabetic foot ulcers are among the most significant complications in people with diabetes mellitus (DM). The number of diabetics is estimated to double by 2030. It is clear that diabetic foot ulcers are a top public healthcare issue. Although the etiology of diabetic foot ulcers remains much unknown, it is widely accepted that repetitive high plantar pressure during walking may initiate the foot ulcer development. Chapter 1, reviews the effects of DM on the changes of composition and structure of the soft tissues of the diabetic foot and how these factors cause abnormally high plantar pressure during walking. Also reviewed are the research methods used to quantify alterations of soft tissue mechanical properties of the diabetic foot. The orthotic devices used in the reduction of peak plantar pressure and healing of diabetic foot ulcers are introduced.

Chapter II - Metallic and non-metallic orthopaedic prostheses have been used widely to replace painful, stiff and mechanically disadvantaged hips. Though the biomaterials used in these implants have been generally considered as inert, adverse tissue reactions in metal-on-polyethylene and more recently metal-on-metal hip arthroplasties have been described since the early 1970s. This can result in premature failure of these implants and need for revision surgery. Recently, a specific implant has been recalled internationally. There has been a worldwide increase in the rate of revision surgery for hip resurfacing arthroplasty due to adverse soft tissue reactions. Inflammatory pseudotumours are a well-described clinical complication of metal-on-metal and recent evidence has suggested similar complications for non-metal-on-metal hip implants. Metal hypersensitivity has been characterized by a predominantly lymphocytic immune response and causes soft-tissue changes such as effusions, pseudotumours and osteolysis. Radiological and histopathological studies have characterized this phenomenon with inflammation, with an emphasis on metal debris as integral to the pathogenesis of this phenomenon. Also, the carcinogenic properties of cadmium, chromium, cobalt, beryllium and other metals utilized in orthopaedic devices have been proven in animal models. This book chapter will discuss the biologic and physical effects of hip athroplasty on soft tissue including pseudotumours and hip arthroplasty-related malignancies.

Chapter 3 - For the orthodontist, orthodontic anchorage has always been a challenge because of tooth movement under the influence of forces applied to them. The use of conventional anchorage (elastic and removable extraoral face-bow) has certain drawbacks for the practitioner and the patient, including full cooperation on the part of that, some degree of discomfort and undesirable side effects. The minimplant can be used for both horizontal and vertical orthodontic traction; they are small enough to fit between the mesial and distal roots of the molars for their intrusion. Placed in the palatal area, these miniscrews can produce sufficient anchorage for molar distalization. Note that miniscrews are too small to cause irreversible bone damage. They can be submitted at any time when the orthodontist or the patient wants and bone healing after removal is done without any incident. These anchoring devices have successes but also failures with particular problems of soft tissue inflammation, problems with patient comfort, the difficulties associated with the development of mechanics and orthodontic appliance on them (springs, chains...), stability problems of anchoring device, and removal. Experimental studies, especially on the animal model, were able to study the various functional and morphological responses of both implants used for orthodontic anchorage (surface geometry), as the surrounding tissue (especially bone surrounding the implant). Various studies have investigated the histological, histo-morphometric and microscopic bone-implant interface. However, the different reactions of the peri-implant tissues, especially soft tissue, are not yet widely studied. Little information is available on the influence of miniscrew on the development and maintenance of the barrier of peri-implant soft tissues. Current knowledge about the barrier of soft tissue is based primarily on animal experiments. However, the results of animal studies do not always correspond to the biological behavior of soft tissue in humans. For practical and ethical reasons, the study in humans is usually subject to differences in the parameters influencing the tissue response such as changes in local conditions of the mucosa, healing time, patient age, smoking and others. In addition, these orthodontics' devices in oral environment are subject to electrochemical corrosion; they may not only generate a progressive biodegradation of the material on the surface, but also of the oxidation process to release potentially allergenic and harmful substances. It is important to note that surface mini-screws tribological properties in orthodontics have been poorly investigated; in addition, their complex approach represent a major "challenge" for orthodontists.

Chapter IV - Temperature related tissue injuries are often present in most hyperthermia treatments. Tissue temperature and its mechanical properties are closely related due to the physiological changes caused by high temperature. An increase in tissue temperature will result in a decrease in moisture content in tissue, and permanent cell necrosis when temperature exceeds a threshold. It is therefore necessary to review the connection between temperature, mechanical properties and injury during hyperthermia treatment. A full understanding between the tissue temperature and mechanical properties allow for possible injury assessment through methods for detecting mechanical properties change such as Magnetic Resonance Elastography (MRE) and vice versa. Many forms of hyperthermia treatment exist in clinical practices; Radiofrequency (RF) ablation, Microwave ablation, Laser ablation, Ultrasonic ablation and Cryo-ablation. This publication concentrates on thermal injury caused by RF ablation and its effects on liver tissue temperature and mechanical properties. RF assisted methods have been widely used in the treatment for hepatocellular cancers, breast tumors and cardiology treatments. RF ablation works on the principle of a high frequency electric current which generates ionic agitation and frictional heating in the target tissue. Catheters used for RF ablation are often needle electrodes for high current density and can be found in two forms; monopolar or bipolar electrodes. Monopolar electrodes work on the principle of a single polarity electrode with a large grounding pad attached to patients while bipolar electrodes are electrode pairs with dual polarity hence do not require a grounding pad. The electric field lines that are induced from the electrode tip by the applied voltage causes an electric force on the charged ions within the electrolytic medium of the liver tissue. This induced force produces a motion that causes ions in the tissue to rub against the surrounding fluid medium, causing friction and thus frictional heating. Increase in tissue temperature due to RF ablation results in moisture loss and protein denaturalization. Moffitt et al. (2002) and Walsh Jr et al (1989) both reported differences in mechanical property between native and thermally damaged liver. In the experiments reviewed, observations were also made for ablation time, to be positively related to a change in tissue stiffness. Ablation time is a good approximation for tissue temperature and hence a relationship can be established between tissue temperature and mechanical properties. Mechanical properties of tissue can be measured by a compression test rig in-vitro or Magnetic Resonance Elastography (MRE) in-vivo. Temperature of tissue sample can be measured by thermocouple for point measurements and thermal cameras for plane measurements. Degree of tissue injury is not only a function of temperature but also a function of time exposed to a critical temperature. Liver tumor necrosis occurs at 45°C when held for long duration (hours) while necrosis occurs within minutes when temperature is above 60°C Hence, tissue injury has to be correlated to temperature and exposed time. The degree of injury can be quantified by means of optical and fluorescence characteristics or Optical Coherence Tomography (OCT). Tissue variation is a big hurdle in the relationship between tissue injury, tissue temperature and mechanical properties. Microstructure variation in liver tissue causes non-systematic temperature distribution due to the many tissue variables; electric conductivity, thermal conductivity, blood perfusion rate, density, etc., governed by Joule heating and bioheat transfer equation. Hence affects homogeneity of RF ablation lesions and mechanical properties. A novel method is required to handle tissue variation for better simulation results and correlation between temperature and mechanical properties. A stochastic model might be a good approach to account for the tissue variation, while nondestructive medical imaging methods such as CT or MRI can be a topographic tool for large vessel placements in correlation models.

Chapter V - Because the cause of musculoskeletal pain can be difficult to determine clinically in many cases, magnetic resonance imaging (MRI) is increasingly utilized to assess the anatomic location, extent and severity of several pathologic conditions offending muscle.MR imaging findings when correlated with clinical features and findings from other methods as electro-myography may facilitate institution of correct diagnosis.Not infrequently, though, the presumptive diagnosis of skeletal muscle disease (myopathy) cannot be made on the basis of clinical- radiologic correlation; and, muscle biopsy is required to ensure diagnosis.Myopathy is suspected when patients complain that the involved muscle is painful and tender, experience difficulty performing tasks that require muscle strength, or develop various systemic manifestations as skin rash or respiratory problems.Infectious, inflammatory, traumatic, neurologic, neoplastic and iatrogenic conditions can cause abnormal signal intensity at MR imaging.Although diverse, some diseases have similar MR imaging appearances, whereas others present distinct patterns of signal intensity abnormality.In general, alterations in muscle signal intensity fall into one of three cardinal patterns: muscle edema, fatty infiltration, and mass lesion.Because some of the muscular disorders, but not all, may require medical or surgical treatment institution of early diagnosis is important.This chapter will review and illustrate the spectrum of MRI appearances in several primary and systemic disorders affecting muscle, both common and uncommon.We believe this work provides a collective —yet succinct and useful guide to a wide array of myopathies.

Chapter VI - The use of bone graft material harvested from the mandibular symphysis to rehabilitate bone defects is considered to be a reliable procedure offering easy access and good quality bone tissue. The literature indicates the suitability of this donor area for reconstructing intra-oral defects with extensions of up to four teeth, and correcting alveolar-palatine clefts and orbital cavity defects. Most studies involving grafts obtained from this donor region are concerned with the characteristics of the bone graft itself rather than the alterations that its removal may cause in adjacent soft tissues or precautions to be taken with them. The authors have sought to make a prospective assessment of neurosensory disturbances, alterations to soft tissue contours and patients' perceptions of the changes occurring after mandibular symphysis bone graft removal. Results show that neurosensory disturbances affect 50% of patients immediately after surgery but as the months go by that percentage reduces considerably. Soft tissue contours are altered by the procedure mainly due to the difficulty of accurately repositioning the mentalis muscles which may lead to an eversion of the lower lip compatible with labial ptosis. Patients report a perception of paresthesia in the operated region and even months afterwards that condition tends to persist However they also declare that the paresthesia does not interfere with eating, speaking or lower lip movements. Another interesting fact is that patients do not notice any alteration to the profile of the operated area. It can be concluded that the use of bone graft material removed from the mandibular symphysis region causes neurosensorial disturbances and alterations to the soft tissue contours but patients declare that those disturbances and alterations do not interfere in their daily routines.

In: Soft Tissue
Editors: A. J. Chavez Ruiz et al.
ISBN 978-1-62257-363-9

Chapter I

Soft Tissue Biomechanics of Diabetic Foot Ulcers

***Chi-Wen Lung*[1,2] *and Yih-Kuen Jan*[2]**
[1]Department of Creative Product Design, Asia University, Taichung, Taiwan, ROC
[2]Department of Rehabilitation Sciences, University of Oklahoma Health Sciences Center, Oklahoma City, Oklahoma, US

Abstract

Diabetic foot ulcers are among the most significant complications in people with diabetes mellitus (DM). The number of diabetics is estimated to double by 2030. It is clear that diabetic foot ulcers are a top public healthcare issue. Although the etiology of diabetic foot ulcers remains much unknown, it is widely accepted that repetitive high plantar pressure during walking may initiate the foot ulcer development. In this chapter, we review the effects of DM on the changes of composition and structure of the soft tissues of the diabetic foot and how these factors cause abnormally high plantar pressure during walking.

We also review research methods used to quantify alterations of soft tissue mechanical properties of the diabetic foot. The orthotic devices used in the reduction of peak plantar pressure and healing of diabetic foot ulcers are introduced.

1. Introduction

Diabetes mellitus (DM) is the seventh leading cause of death by disease in the United States [1]. The classification of DM proposed by the World Health Organization (WHO) includes four categories, including insulin-dependent diabetes mellitus (IDDM), noninsulin-dependent diabetes mellitus (NIDDM), malnutrition-related diabetes mellitus (MRDM), and other types of diabetes associated with certain conditions and syndromes [2].

DM is recognized by chronic elevation of the concentration of glucose in the blood (hyperglycemia), which may cause many complications, including heart diseases, blindness, kidney failure, diabetic foot ulcers and related amputations [3]. Regarding diabetic foot ulcers, it is estimated that 15% of diabetics will develop a foot ulcer during their lifetime [4], and 2-3% of the population may develop a foot ulcer annually [5]. The total cost associated with treating a diabetic foot ulcer is about $13,179 [6], for a total of $58 billion in the United States [7]

The human foot is a unique structure in the animal kingdom, as it is capable of supporting sustained bipedal gait. The plantar soft tissues, especially in the forefoot and heel regions, are specially structured to provide functions of cushioning and shock absorption to protect the underlying tissues and support the body in general during locomotion activities [8]. Alterations in foot biomechanics caused by changes in the properties of soft tissue have been postulated as a key risk factor for the diabetic foot ulcers [9]. DM causes thickening and stiffening of collagen rich tissues, which may lead to an abnormally high plantar pressure [10].

The high plantar pressure together with diabetic peripheral neuropathy [11, 12], previous foot trauma, or foot deformities [11] may contribute to diabetic foot ulcerations.

In addition to the neuropathic and vascular components, the alterations in morphology (such as Charcot foot) and structure (such as hammer/claw toes) also occur in the diabetic foot. The foot injury that initiates ulcers could result either from trauma or from a repetitive mechanical stress [13].

Diabetic foot ulcers are more common at the forefoot under the first and second metatarsal heads as compared to the heels [14, 15]. For diabetics, local stiffness in proximity of the first metatarsal head is substantially larger than in other sites, and this could be associated with initial tissue ulceration at this location [16]. Klaesner and colleagues [17] showed that the plantar tissue over the metatarsal head in diabetics with peripheral neuropathy was significantly stiffer than age-matched control subjects. Armstrong et al. [18] found the locations of ulcers in twenty-five consecutive diabetics with neuropathic foot ulcers were hallux (4%), first to fifth metatarsal head (52%, 12%, 8%, 0%, and 12%, respectively), lateral midfoot (4%), and heel (8%), and concluded the first metatarsal head is the most common site of diabetic foot ulcers. Previous studies have shown that plantar tissue properties vary by location [19] that may contribute to a higher incidence rate of foot ulcers in certain plantar locations [20].

Several diabetic foot ulcer classification systems have been proposed. However, these classifications are based on neuropathy, arteriopathy, and geometric ulcer size, they do not consider the role of the soft tissue mechanical properties of the diabetic foot.

The foot ulcers usually occur in the plantar side. The six-grade Wagner-Meggitt classification [21] used for decades classifies wounds by the depth of ulceration and extent of gangrene. The system [21] grades wound by depth and then stages them by the presence or absence of infection and ischemia, but it does not include neuropathy or ulcer location. Five categories include size (area, depth), sepsis, arteriopathy, and denervation (SAD) with classification grades on a four-point scale (0- 3) [22].

Similarly, the International Working Group of the Diabetic Foot (IWGDF) proposed five features including perfusion (arterial supply), extent (area), depth, infection, and sensation (PEDIS) in the classification [23], which grades the wound. The Infectious Diseases Society of America published a guideline [24] to classify infected diabetic foot wounds into the categories of mild (restricted involvement of only skin and subcutaneous tissues), moderate (more extensive or affecting deeper tissues), and severe (accompanied by systemic signs of infection or metabolic instability).

Structural soft tissue changes in the diabetic foot of neuropathic patients, in terms of bone and muscle density, joint angle and arthropathy, and plantar soft tissue thickness, have also been revealed as causative factors of foot ulcers [25].

As the incidence of DM is increasing globally, diabetic foot ulcer has become a top public health issue. A better understanding of diabetic foot biomechanics may improve the evaluation and treatment of diabetic foot ulcers [26-28].

2. Internal Contributors to Diabetic Foot Ulcerations

The abnormal plantar pressure generated during walking causes most diabetic foot ulcers. Higher plantar pressure is associated with changes of composition and structure of diabetic foot soft tissues. We describe the changes of soft tissues of the diabetic foot in two categories, composition and structural changes and mechanical properties of soft tissues of the diabetic foot.

2.1. Composition and Structural Changes of Diabetic Foot Soft Tissues

DM affects connective tissues in many ways and causes different alterations in the periarticular and skeletal systems. Musculoskeletal disorders are common in diabetics, and examination of periarticular regions of the hands, the joints, shoulders and feet, as well as the skeleton, should be included in the evaluation [29].

2.1.1. Foot Deformities

Hyperglycemia induces metabolic derangements that directly affect the Schwann cells (myelin) and nodes of Ranvier (axons). Hyperglycemia may also affect the structure and function of endoneurial microvessels, thereby altering the blood-nerve barrier and causing local hypoxia or ischemia [30]. This may lead to peripheral sensory neuropathy, which evolves in about 25% of adult diabetic patients [31]. Peripheral neuropathy induces foot deformities in diabetics. The changed appearance will happen in the diabetic foot, which includes hammer/claw toes, hallux valgus, hallux limitus, prominent metatarsal heads, bony prominences, Charcot deformity, plantar callus, foot type (a broad spectrum ranging from pes cavus or high arch feet to neutrally aligned or normal arch feet to pes planus or low arch feet), muscle atrophy, ankle and hallux mobility [20, 32]. Due to excessive localized pressures on insensitive skin, foot deformities could be a possible risk factor for diabetic foot ulcerations [11].

The foot deformities are induced by the diabetic peripheral neuropathy on the soft tissues. For example, hammer/claw toes [33]; the main function of the toes in gait is to contact the surface and exert sufficient pressure to obtain a fixed point from which the body can be propelled. This way, the toes help to relieve the metatarsal head from bearing weight through the distal transfer of load in the final stage before push-off. The toes in the neuropathic subjects with deformity have become less functional by showing a significantly reduced contact area and force-time integral when compared with the toes of the controls. With less functional toes, the metatarsal head bears an increased amount of weight during propulsion as evidenced by the significant reduction in the toe-loading index found in the patients with deformity. These findings confirm suggestions by Boulton et al. [34] that the presence of claw/hammer toes may be responsible for the lower toe-loading ratio found in diabetic groups compared with non-diabetics. Thus, while the fat pad migrates distally in the foot [35], the load migrates proximally in the foot, a process called the fat pad-plantar pressure exchange principle. Morag and Cavanagh [36] established foot structure and function predicted only approximately 50% of the variance in peak pressure, although the relative contributions in different anatomical regions varied dramatically. Mueller and colleagues [37] used parameters derived from computed tomography (CT) scans to predict up to 71% of the variance in peak plantar pressure in diabetic neuropathic subjects and up to 83% for non-diabetics. Other studies found that certain deformities increase the peak pressure in the forefoot and toes [33, 38]. Recent imaging data have shown that there is a physiologic relation to increased pressure in the forefoot due to hammer/claw toe deformity [35]. However, Cowley and colleagues [20] showed that certain foot deformities were predictive of ulceration, although there was no relationship between the clinical foot deformity and ulcer location.

Foot deformities are not necessarily linked to a specific location of ulceration [20]. Once diabetes has progressed to a certain point, other factors may become more influential on ulcer location, such as peripheral neuropathy, peripheral vascular disease, skin deterioration and abnormal mechanical trauma (acute injury). Perhaps, if no other factors were involved, these deformities on their own could cause ulceration by inducing long periods of repetitive stress on the soft tissues of the foot [20].

2.1.2. Limited Joint Mobility

DM has been recognized to cause a wide range of musculoskeletal disorders, including tenosynovitis, joint stiffness, and tendon contracture. Several possible biochemical abnormalities related to disturbances in glucose metabolism may contribute to limited joint mobility [29]. One of the diabetic syndromes is hyperglycemia, which promotes glycosilation of proteins and the consequent accumulation of AGE in most human tissues [39]. Since the 1950s, it has been clinically observed that the abnormal AGE storage of collagenous layers in the tissue could be thickening of tendinous and ligamentous structures of diabetic foot [40]. This means these soft tissues, including muscles, cartilages, tendons, and ligaments, may experience structural changes even before the onset of diabetic neuropathy.

The thickness of plantar fascia is directly correlated with vertical forces under the metatarsal heads. In diabetic patients, soft tissue involvement may contribute to the increase of vertical forces under the metatarsal heads. Changes in the structure of plantar fascia may also influence the mobility of the first metatarso-phalangeal joint [41]. Moreover, thickening of plantar fascia and Achilles tendon in diabetics is more evident in the presence of neuropathy, which poorly absorbs shock during the gait (performs the physiological impact force absorption during the gait). More generally, an overall alteration of the ankle joint motion likely occurs throughout the whole gait cycle, which partly explains the abnormal loading under the forefoot [42]. The maximum frontal plane ankle joint moment was smaller in the neuropathic diabetic subjects in the walking pattern [43]. Limited joint mobility (LJM) of the ankle joint is associated with increased peak forefoot pressures [44], and therefore mechanical stress has been recognized to have a central pathogenic role in the onset of diabetic neuropathic ulcers [45].

Not only could the connective tissues be affected of LJM of the foot and ankle efficiency in gait, but also the muscle. The electromyography (EMG) responses of the thigh and leg muscles in the diabetic neuropathic group were delayed if compared to the normal recruitment pattern, especially the tibialis anterior and vastus lateralis. The peripheral diabetic neuropathy causes impairments in not only somatosensorial and motor sources but also intrinsic mechanisms of motor control leading to alterations in the ankle efficiency in gait [46]. The midfoot and forefoot play a different role in people with neuropathy by receiving higher loads at push-off phase that are probably due to smaller ankle flexion at the stance phase [47].

2.1.3. Skin Thickness Changes

The epidermal layer of diabetic foot becomes thinner and plantar soft tissues become stiffer in diabetics, particularly in persons with neuropathy or ulceration [48]. However, in another study, the plantar epidermal thickness was significantly thicker in type 2 diabetics without neuropathy compared with non-diabetics [49]. The total thickness of plantar soft tissues should be considered as a whole when it serves as the cushion for optimizing load-bearing during walking. However, the total plantar soft tissue thickness is composed of various layers of tissues including the skin (dermis and epidermis), fat pads, fascia, and muscle. The evidence suggests that the process of injury in diabetic feet may not initiate entirely on the skin surface, but also in deeper plantar soft tissue layers [50, 51]. The morphology of the skin is composed of an outer thinner epidermal and an inner thicker dermal layer [52]. However, research showed that pure type 2 diabetics tend to have thicker epidermis/skin of the foot as compared to non-diabetics. In contrast, epidermal thinning of plantar skin occurs in people who have clinical manifestations of diabetic neuropathy and ulceration. On the other hand, the total thickness and stiffness of plantar soft tissue were increased in all people with diabetes, in which a greater increase was found in diabetics with neuropathy and ulceration. Such a decrease in the epidermal thickness of plantar skin, but an increase in the stiffness of total plantar soft tissue, makes the diabetic foot prone to tissue breakdown and hence ulcer formation [48].

Bus et al. [35] showed that the fat pads in the plantar tissues of diabetic peripheral neuropathy subjects with toe deformities were significantly thinner under the metatarsal head but thicker under the phalanges. They postulated that this alteration in fat pad thickness could be due to the distal movement of fat pads caused by toe deformities. Compared with the control group, the average epidermal thickness of plantar skin was reduced by 15% in people with diabetic foot ulceration and 9% in people with neuropathy, but was increased by 6% in pure diabetics.

Previous work on the diabetic foot has examined the thickness of different tissues such as the plantar fascia [41]. They found an increase in both the thickness of the plantar fascia and the vertical forces under the metatarsal head in people with diabetes (who may or may not have neuropathy). The soft tissues on specific plantar pressure points for diabetic neuropathy in elderly people were significantly stiffer and thinner than that of the healthy young people [53]. Duffin and colleagues [54] reported that the plantar aponeurosis was significantly thicker in young diabetics, and conversely the skin thickness was not significantly different.

Robertson and colleagues [25] did not find significant differences in the plantar soft tissue thickness beneath the metatarsal heads between people with diabetes and healthy controls. They suggested that alterations in the glycation of plantar epidermal proteins may change the thickness of the plantar skin or epidermis. In the diabetic heel pad, tissue properties are altered heterogeneously in people with diabetes [55]. We summarize the skin thickness between diabetics and no-diabetics from previous studies in Table 1.

Table 1. Comparison of epidermis/skin thickness between diabetics and non-diabetics

Study	Thicker in diabetics	Thinner in diabetics	No differences between diabetics and non-diabetics
Chao et al., 2011 [48].	plantar epidermis in pure type 2 diabetes	plantar epidermis in diabetic neuropathy and ulceration	--
Bus et al., 2004 [35]	under the phalanges in diabetic neuropathy	metatarsal head in diabetic neuropathy	--
Bus et al., 2004 [35]	plantar epidermis in diabetic foot ulceration and neuropathy	plantar epidermis in pure diabetes	--
D'Ambrogi et al., 2003 [41]	plantar fascia in diabetes (who may or may not have neuropathy)	--	--
Duffin et al., 2002 [54]	--	--	plantar skin in type 1 diabetes
Robertson et al., 2002 [25]	--	--	plantar skin in diabetes
Hashmi et al., 2006 [49]	plantar epidermis in type 2 diabetes without neuropathy	--	--
Zheng et al., 2000 [53]	--	plantar skin in elder diabetics with neuropathy	--

2.2. Mechanical Properties of Diabetic Foot Soft Tissues

DM causes abnormal collagen deposition in the periarticular connective tissues that alters the structural and the mechanical properties of soft tissues [29]. Several observations pointed to alterations of collagen structure and function in diabetics [10, 56, 57]. A number of studies identified alterations in collagen structure and function as related to the glucose-exposure. The process of nonenzymatic glycosylation (NEG) may play a significant role in the development of chronic complications of diabetes [58].

Diabetic skin consistently stained more intensely for glucitollysine than non-diabetic skin. Antigens present in both the epidermis and the eccrine structures reacted with the antibody in both diabetic and non-diabetic skin but with greater intensity in the diabetic skin.

Formation of advanced glycation end products (AGE) has been shown to be associated with the structural alterations of long-lived matrix components, such as cross-linking of adjacent collagen fibrils [59]. Glucose exposure causes changes in the mechanical properties of collagenous tissues supported by both *in vitro* [60] and animal [61] studies. The altered properties of connective tissues includes increased fibril diameter, closer packing of fibrils and irregular fibril shapes (indicating local fusion of adjacent fibrils). The AGE inhibitor aminoguanidine (AG) has been shown to reduce AGE accumulation and significantly inhibit several vascular and renal manifestations in diabetics [62]. In addition, AG treatments reduced AGE-related changes of the biophysical properties of connective tissue, such as increase in collagen stability of rats with experimental diabetes [63].

The changes in tissue stiffness can be quantified by the elastic (E) component in the Kelvin-Voight viscoelastic model. Diabetes causes substantial stiffening of the affected tissues, including hyperkeratosis and formation of thickened callus in the plantar skin [64]. The stiffness of plantar soft tissue tends to increase in all diabetic groups compared with non-diabetics [48, 65]. This mechanism has an overall effect of mechanically stiffening the plantar tissues [16, 66]. Hence, the overall cushioning property of the plantar soft tissue, especially at high-pressure sites such as those under the medial metatarsals, is reduced.

The tissue energy dissipation ratio can be quantified by the viscous (η) component as the hysteresis of non-linear damper in Kelvin-Voight viscoelastic model. Hsu and colleagues [67] provided an ultrasound transducer mounted on the loading-unloading device conducted to simulate the heel pad stress-strain relationship in the loaded and unloaded states. A transmission electron microscope was used to examine the heel specimens taken from amputated legs in diabetics and non-diabetics. They found the diabetic patients had a significantly higher mean energy dissipation ratio, and the collagen fibrils in diabetic heel samples were ruptured with unclear striation and uneven distribution. Gefen and colleagues [66] showed that the stress-strain relation of the heel pad was highly non-linear, the compression modulus was 105 kPa initially and 306 kPa at 30% strain. The energy dissipation during heel strike was evaluated to be 17.8%. The curvature parameters may explain the poor rebound phenomenon resulting in the high impact energy in diabetic heel pads. Breakdown in collagen fibrils may be responsible for this observation.

Caballero and colleagues [68] assessed endothelium-dependent and endothelium-independent responses in skin microcirculation. The responses to both acetylcholine chloride (ACh) and sodium nitroprusside (SNP) were reduced in the diabetic groups compared with controls. It is known that ACh stimulates nitric oxide production in endothelial cells (endothelium-dependent vasodilation). Endothelial dysfunction is one of the primary pathways that lead to nerve hypoxia and to the development of diabetic neuropathy. Diabetic neuropathy itself has an additional detrimental effect on the foot microcirculation [69]. The final result of all the above changes is that the diabetic foot fails to mount a satisfactory hyperemic response to injury and is susceptible to ulceration and/or impaired wound healing [70]. As most neuropathic diabetic patients need to use moisturizing cream for the dry skin of the lower extremity, the addition of a vasodilator that will increase the blood flow may prove of particular help [71].

2.2.1. Indentation Tests

In 1912, Schade developed an indentation apparatus to study the creep properties of skin and the changes that result from edematous conditions [72]. Since then, several indentation methods have been developed in the past decades to characterize the mechanical properties of the thickness or stiffness of plantar soft tissue. The medical imaging methods including magnetic resonance imaging (MRI), X-ray, optical coherence tomography, and ultrasound have been used for this purpose [73]. Horikawa and colleagues [74] also used a laser distance sensor to determine the indentation depth. The main difference of these methods comes from the techniques to measure the displacement of the indenter or the deformation of tissues. The indenter was driven either manually [74-76] or pneumatically [77, 78] onto the skin surface. The most popular technique for determining the *in vivo* biomechanical behaviors of soft tissues is the indentation test. The test itself very much resembles that of palpation of the plantar soft tissues [53, 65].

The portability of these systems is always a problem for *in vivo* operations with a bulk measurement device. In order to solve this problem, Zheng and colleagues [75] have developed a hand-held tissue ultrasound palpation system (TUPS) that utilizes a single ultrasound transducer in tandem with a load cell to measure the stiffness of plantar soft tissues in healthy controls and people with diabetes (Figures 1 and 2). The diabetic foot of the tissue thickness can also be obtained with ultrasound measurements [48, 65]. Therefore, ultrasound indentation has become one of the most popular indentation techniques in recent decades to measure the mechanical properties of plantar soft tissues with its capability of real-time imaging function. The system comprises a pen-size probe having an ultrasound transducer at the tip and a load cell connected in series with it.

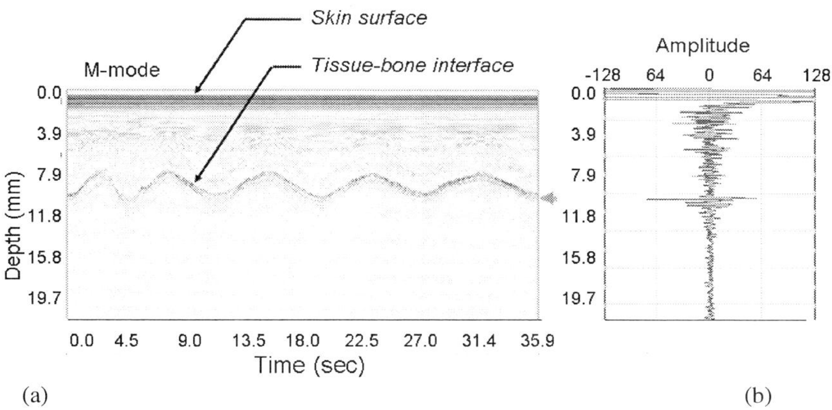

Figure 1. An example of indentation data from the tissue ultrasound palpation system (TUPS). (a) It shows the ultrasound echo trains. The first echo is associated with the ultrasound transducer-skin interface while the second one represents the tissue-bone interface. The thickness of the heel pad is presented by the distance between the first and second echoes. (b) The cross-section of the heel tissues corresponding to the echoes obtained by TUPS for measuring thickness.

Recently TUPS was used to study the thickness and **Young's** modulus of plantar soft tissues in people are reported in Tables 2 and 3 [48, 53, 65, 73, 79, 80].

2.2.2. Viscoelastic Models

Several biomechanical models have been used to characterize the viscoelastic properties of the diabetic foot. The Kelvin-Voight viscoelastic model [66] and quasi-linear viscoelastic (QLV) models [19, 81, 82] are used for assessing the property of plantar soft tissues.

The Kelvin-Voight viscoelastic model, with linearly elastic spring in parallel to a non-linear damper, is similarly representing the stress-strain characteristics of the plantar soft tissue (Figure 3).

Gefen and colleagues [66] used the following viscoelastic constitutive law to describe the *in vivo* stress-strain behavior of the human heel pad during gait:

$$\sigma_c = -E\varepsilon_c - \eta\varepsilon_c\dot{\varepsilon}_c \qquad \text{Eq. (1)}$$

The heel-ground contact stress (σ_c) was calculated for each contact pressure display frame by averaging the contact stresses measured in each optical sensor under the heel-ground contact region; the contact stress (σ_c)

versus the heel pad compression strain (ε_c) values. The η and E are the viscous and elastic, respectively.

Table 2. The thickness of plantar soft tissues

		Tissue Thickness, mm			
		1st metatarsal head		Heel	
Study		Normal	DM	Normal	DM
Chao et al., 2010	[79]	12.7(2.1)	--	12.7(2.1)	--
Kwan et al., 2010	[80]	9.2(2.8)	--	20.9 (1.8)	--
Zheng et al., 2000	[53]	12.0(2.0)	6.5(1.0) DM	16.0(1.0)	12.0(2.0) DM
Sun et al., 2011	[65]	7.8(0.4)	8.3(0.3) DPN	18.9(0.7)	18.3(0.5) DPN
Chao et al., 2011	[48]	9.4(1.9)	8.6(1.2) DU	23.7(3.3)	25.1(3.1) DU
Zheng et al., 2011	[73]	--	--	13.8(2.5)	--

Note: DM Diabetic mellitus; DPN Diabetic peripheral neuropathy; DU Diabetic foot ulceration.

Table 3. The Young's modulus of plantar soft tissues

		Young's Modulus, kPa			
		1st metatarsal head		Heel	
Study		Normal	DM	Normal	DM
Chao et al., 2010	[79]	32.9(14.4)	--	--	--
Kwan et al., 2010	[80]	36.8(11.6)	--	32.4(11.9)	--
Zheng et al., 2000	[53]	40.0(15.0)	120.0(50) DM	40.0(5.0)	50(20) DM
Sun et al., 2011	[65]	62.1(9.4)	96.3(7.4) DPN	45.0(4.2)	65.6(4.1) DPN
Chao et al., 2011	[48]	80.1(34.0)	107.1(33.4) DU	69.8(19.8)	87.6(21.4) DU
Zheng et al., 2011	[73]	--	--	40.0(20.7)	--

Note: DM Diabetic mellitus; DPN Diabetic peripheral neuropathy; DU Diabetic foot ulceration.

Gefen and colleagues [66] showed a compression of 40% of the original thickness in 150 ms during initial contact in the heel. The stress-strain relation of the heel pad was shown to be highly non-linear, with a compression modulus of 105±11kPa initially and 306±16kPa at 30% strain.

The energy dissipation during heel strike was evaluated to be 17.8±0.8%. The Kelvin-Voight viscoelastic model is useful for biomechanical as well as clinical evaluation of the stress-strain and energy absorption characteristics of the plantar *in vivo*.

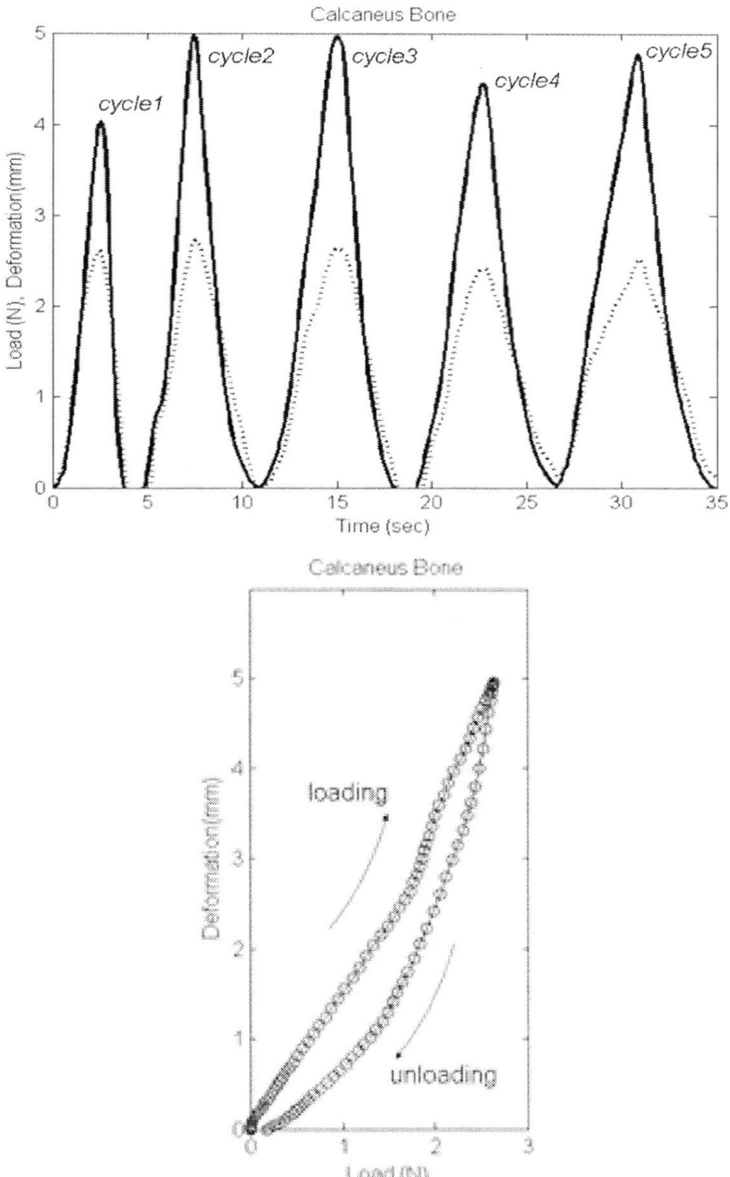

(a)

(b)

Figure 2. Indentation curves and loading-unloading curves of the plantar soft tissues. (a) Five load-indentation curves of Heel, solid line is load force, dotted line is the deformation. (b) Force-deformation curves for the cycle 3 of the heel.

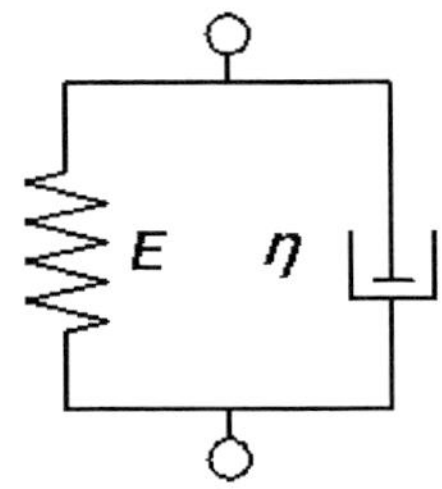

Figure 3. Viscous (η) and elastic (E) properties of Kelvin-Voigt viscoelastic model.

Hayes et al. [83] presented a rigorous mathematical solution to the elasticity problem of indentation of a thin, elastic, homogenous layer of material bonded to a rigid half-space. The solution yields an expression for calculation of the Young's modulus from the indentation load deformation data:

$$E = \frac{1 - v2}{2a\kappa(v, a/h)} \frac{P}{W} \qquad \text{Eq. (2)}$$

In the equation, E is the Young's modulus; P is the applied force; W is the indention depth; a presets the radius of the indenter, v is the Poisson's ratio; h is the tissue thickness; k is a scaling factor which is a function of v and a/h.

Fung's QLV model is a widely used viscoelastic model that provides meaningful phenomenological fit coefficients [84], and has previously been applied to many plantar soft tissues [19, 81, 82].

The basic premise of this theory is that the strain-dependent and time-dependent properties are separable as defined by an elastic function that yields elastic coefficients and a reduced relaxation function that yields viscous coefficients. To address the creep-indentation behavior of articular cartilage, Fung [84] proposed a QLV model to describe the load-deformation relationship of biological soft tissues.

$$T(t) = \int_{-\infty}^{t} G(t-\xi) \cdot \frac{\partial T^{e}(u(\xi))}{\partial u(\xi)} \cdot \frac{\partial u(\xi)}{\partial \xi} \cdot d\xi \qquad \text{Eq. (3)}$$

In this theory, the load response, $T(t)$, of a tissue to an applied deformation history, $u(t)$, was expressed in terms of a convolution integral of a reduced relaxation function $G(t)$, and a nonlinear elastic function $Te(u)$.

If the viscosity of soft tissue is taken into account, an instantaneous Young's modulus in the QLV form is written as [84],

$$E(u,t)=E^{(e)}(u)\ G(t) \qquad \text{Eq. (4)}$$

where $E^{(e)}(u)$ is the un-relaxed elastic modulus and G(t) is the reduced relaxation function for which $G(0 = 1$. For the sake for simplicity, these two functions are proposed as the following forms in this study, i.e.,

$$E^{(e)}(u)= E_0+E_1u \qquad \text{Eq. (5)}$$

$$G(t)= 1- a +\alpha e^{-t/\tau} \qquad \text{Eq. (6)}$$

where E_0 is the initial modulus, E_1 is the non-linear factor, τ is the time constant and α is the viscosity-related constant.

The QLV model was used to estimate the plantar soft tissue properties with stress relaxation experiments *in vitro* [19], and the load-indentation responses were obtained using an ultrasound indentation apparatus with a hand-held pen-sized probe *in vivo* [81]. However, as the result of QLV model *in vitro* by Pai and Ledoux [82], the stress relaxation responses of both diabetic and non-diabetic specimens were similar and accordingly few of the QLV parameters for either fit the approach and none of the raw data parameters differed. Likewise, no differences were found between plantar locations in diabetics.

2.2.3. Finite Element Models

The mechanical interactions between the foot and supportive surfaces can be studied both experimentally and numerically. Recent studies have used the finite element models (FEM) to predict the loading of the foot's components during standing and walking as they relate to foot disorders and therapeutic footwear. FEM is a well-established method for obtaining biomechanical characteristics of the foot, including internal deformation and stress in its skeletal, ligamenteous, muscular, fat and other soft tissue components, a preliminary three-dimensional finite element analysis [85]. X-ray, fluoroscopy, ultrasound, CT, and MRI, all have potential to quantify diabetes-associated changes of the foot. When combined with a device capable of applying known loads to the limb during imaging, these techniques may be used to investigate the internal stress/strain distribution within the foot [86]. A computational model revealed significant tension stress concentrations (90-150 kPa) in the plantar pad of the simulated diabetic forefoot. They were four times the normal maximum stress under the first metatarsal head and almost eight times the normal maximum stress under the second metatarsal head [50].

Patil et al. [87] used a two-dimensional (2-D) model that had been constructed according to a lateral X-ray image in order to study stress distributions in normal and neuropathic feet. Furthermore, fluoroscopy has been used with a plantar-pressure monitoring device to provide real-time dynamic imaging of foot deformation [66]. Subjects walked upon a gait platform integrating the contact pressure display optical method for plantar pressure measurements and a digital radiographic fluoroscopy system for skeletal and soft tissue motion recording. To allow such real-time subject-specific analysis, combined the pressure device and fluoroscopy, it can simultaneous measurements of the plantar pad tissue deformation and the heel-ground contact stresses developing during the stance phase of gait [85]. Yarnitzky et al. [85] developed a hierarchal modeling system which integrates a 2-D gross structural model of the foot with local FEM of the plantar tissue padding. The FEM provides real-time analytical evaluations of the time-dependent plantar pad forces during the stance phase. Unfortunately, poor contrast between different types of soft tissue limits fluoroscopy to imaging the motion of bones within the soft tissue envelope. Fluoroscopy is also a transmission technique that creates 2-D projections of three-dimensional (3-D) structures, making it difficult to reconstruct deformations in closely spaced discrete structures, such as the tissue underneath the metatarsal heads. This is a developed method that combined spiral x-ray CT imaging and plantar pressure analysis to quantify internal foot structure and external pressure during diabetic foot plantar loading [88]. In their studies of the diabetic foot, it applied a total vertical load of 50% of body weight with the foot fixed in 15° of plantar flexion to simulate the late stance phase of walking.

Ultrasound has been used alone to determine the thickness of the forefoot fat pad during standing [89] and walking [90]. In combination with a force measurement device, ultrasound was used to measure the mechanical response of the human heel pad [91]. Erdemir and colleagues [91] used M-mode ultrasound to measure the initial tissue thickness and deformation; indentation forces were recorded simultaneously. An inverse finite-element analysis of the indentation protocol using axisymmetric models adjusted to reflect individual heel thickness was used to extract nonlinear material properties describing the hyperelastic behavior of each heel. Ultrasound is relatively inexpensive and portable, but its utility is restricted by depth limitations, shadowing by bones, and relatively poor contract between soft tissues.

Gefen [50] used the MRI to obtain the geometric data of the foot of an adult female and transferred it to a commercial FEM analysis software package (ANSYS, Inc., Canonsburg, PA, USA) for construction of planar models for the five rays of the foot. The von Mises equivalent stress, $\sigma_{V.M.}$, weighs the effects of principal tension (σ_1) and principal compression (σ_2) stresses according to the relation:

$$\sigma_{V.M.} =. (\sigma_1^2 + \sigma_2^2 + \sigma_1\sigma_2)^{1/2} \qquad \text{Eq. (7)}$$

It was shown that with increased degree of stiffness of the plantar pad, as related to glucose-exposure, peak forefoot contact stresses may raise by 38% and 50% under the first and second metatarsal heads, respectively. The increase in averaged (von Mises) internal stresses within the plantar soft tissues is even more pronounced, and may rise by 82% and 307% for the tissue under the first and second metatarsal heads, respectively. These results, which conform to experimental data gathered over the last two decades, suggest that the process of injury in diabetic feet is very likely to initiate not from the skin surface, but in deeper tissue layers, and the tissues underlying the distal bony prominences of the medial metatarsals are the most vulnerable ones.

3. External Contributors to Diabetic Foot Ulcerations

Several mechanical factors may contribute in various ways to diabetic foot ulcers, including compression (pressure, pressure gradient) and shear (shear stress).

3.1. Plantar Pressure

Abnormally high plantar pressure, together with neuropathy and altered compositions of soft tissues of the diabetic, are the main risk factors causing foot ulceration, which may lead to amputation of the lower extremity in diabetics [27, 92]. This mechanism has an overall effect of mechanically stiffening the plantar tissues, especially if high-pressure sites such as those under the medial metatarsals is damaged. Foot deformity or displacement of soft tissues can lead to high plantar pressure [15, 93] and failure to heal [94]. Pressure between the foot and ground at a bony prominence can exceed 1,000 kPa, whereas pressure between a correctly applied total contact cast and a potential ulcer site is less than 100 kPa [95]. Peak plantar pressure has been investigated extensively in the literature as a surrogate measure of trauma to the plantar foot and is known to be an important contributing factor to skin breakdown in diabetics with peripheral neuropathy [15, 93, 96]. During barefoot walking, forefoot pressures are much higher than rearfoot pressures (forefoot-to-rearfoot pressure ratio 2.3±2.4 in subjects with diabetes and severe neuropathy [15]. While walking in shoes, however, peak plantar pressure under the forefoot tends to be similar to that in the rearfoot (242±25 kPa in the forefoot compared with 240±28 kPa in the rearfoot) [96].

3.2. Plantar Pressure Gradient

Plantar shear forces are probably important, but cannot be easily measured at present. Mueller and colleagues [97] used the pressure sensor to describe another variable, peak pressure gradient (PPG), the value between the adjacent regions of the peak plantar pressure (PPP) that appears to provide additional information regarding the potential trauma to the foot's soft tissues. As one simple example, underwater divers experience very high hydrostatic pressures; however, these pressures do not result in skin breakdown because the high pressures are distributed evenly across the surface of their skin. The large pressure gradients could contribute to skin breakdown because they generate large shearing stresses within the soft tissues.

A normal pressure load on the plantar surface may be characterized by the PPP and PPG. The PPP is defined as

$$PPP = max\,(p) \qquad \text{Eq. (8)}$$

where p is the pressure distribution on the plantar surface. The PPG at the PPP location can be calculated by

$$PPG = \max\left(\frac{\partial p}{\partial r} \bigg|_{(x_p, y_p)} \right) \qquad \text{Eq. (9)}$$

where $\left(\left.\frac{\partial p}{\partial r}\right|_{(x_p,y_p)}\right)$ (space rate of change of pressure on the plantar surface) is the directional derivative of pressure P at the PPP location (x_p, y_p) on the plantar surface in any direction given by vector $\vec{r}$.

Zou et al. [98] showed in forefoot and rearfoot, the PPP ratio was 136% (371 kPa and 272 kPa), but the PPG ratio was increased 243% (34 kPa/mm and 14 kPa/mm). PPG may perhaps be more discriminating than peak plantar pressure alone in distinguishing between groups of individuals who are at risk for diabetic foot ulcers [99]. The peak pressure and the PPG obtained from the interface pressure distribution appear to be important variables to identify where maximum shear stress are located in the subsurface tissues on the plantar foot that may lead to skin break down [98].

3.3. Shear Stress

Veves et al. [93] showed that only 38% of diabetic foot ulcers developed under the area where the peak pressure was found at the first visit. Lavery and colleagues [100] suggested that pressure cannot be the sole factor associated with development of skin breakdown. There should be other factors at play that increase predictive potential when combined with plantar foot pressure assessment. Shear stress may be an important factor in locating where skin breakdown occurs in patients at high risk for ulceration. The shear stress tends to make the foot slip from its relatively fixed position on the ground during walking. This shear stress generates separately in the tissues and the shoe materials. Since 1992, a miniature triaxial force transducer (4.9 x 16 mm diameter) has been developed to measure plantar shear stress [101]. Lord and colleagues [102] used a bi-axial magneto-resistive shear transducer, and the diabetic group exhibited lower magnitudes of shear stress under the third/fourth metatarsal heads (average 51/39 vs. 86.5/71 kPa, respectively) and higher magnitudes under the first/second heads (73/64 vs. 35/31 kPa, respectively), indicating a medial shift. Step-to-step variability of maximum shear measured under the third metatarsal head showed an increase in the transverse component.

Akhlaghi and Pepper [103] used piezoelectric film for the independent measurements of the three orthogonal components of force, the authors found the peak shear force values were between 16% and 75% of peak vertical forces. Yavuz and colleagues [104-106] used a custom-built shear and pressure platform, 80 sensors (12.5mm x 12.5mm) arranged in an 8x10 array to collect local barefoot forces acting on the foot-ground interface. Their result [106] described that the people walking yielded the antero-posterior and medio-lateral shear stresses which were 76.1 and 50.9 kPa, respectively. A predicted peak antero-posterior shear stress magnitude was as high as 97.8 kPa. The authors [104] found shear-time integral values were increased in the diabetic group by 61% and 132% for AP and resultant shear cases, respectively. They also found [105] diabetic subject's representative peak stress profiles, where the peak pressure occurred under the second metatarsal head, whereas the peak shear was under the hallux. Stucke and colleagues [107] used 400 x 580 x 1.7 mm surface stress sensitive film. The average peak shear values were higher in the forefoot than in the heel. This study suggested that the interactions of the shear forces caused greater "spreading" in the forefoot and greater tissue "dragging" in the heel. The results also showed that peak shear stresses do not occur at the same site or time as peak pressure. All of these devices are currently being used only in research environments.

Cong et al. [108] used a triaxial force transducer (10 x 17 mm diameter, Bioforcen, Inc., Hefei, Anhui, China). They found the peak resultant shear was the largest at the hallux (12.9 kPa) for the heel height of 30 mm shoes during balanced standing by healthy people. These studies measured shear stress range on the plantar aspect of human feet, which indicated that the diacritic foot could have significantly higher shear stress. In this regard, plantar shear has the potential to fill gaps in our understanding of the complex etiology of plantar soft tissue ulceration.

4. Diabetic Foot Ulcer Healing and Prevention

The treatment of diabetic foot ulcers includes infection control, wound care (debridement), wound surgery (revascularization), supportive treatment (off-loading and protecting), adjuvant treatment (antibiotics, oxygen therapy), and amputation [3, 109]. It is important to evaluate whether diabetic peripheral neuropathy or peripheral vascular disease is present [26]. Simple surgery like split skin grafting or minor toe amputations may be necessary and complex surgery like flap coverage is indicated for younger diabetics with foot ulcers. The merits of an intact lower limb with an abnormal foot have to be weighed against amputation and prosthesis in the overall planning of limb salvage or sacrifice [109]. If limb salvage is the decision, additional means like oxygen therapy, and other alternative medicines, might have benefits. The off-loading of footwear should always be a major consideration as a prevention of ulcer formation [109].

During weight-bearing activities, the feet are exposed to large forces, particularly when the activity is dynamic, such as walking. Increased plantar pressures and associated ulcers need to be treated by off-loading of the plantar surface. The off-loading of footwear should always be a major consideration as a prevention of ulcer formation. These plantar off-loading mechanisms could result in an optimization of treatment, but clinical effectiveness must be demonstrated. While this is far superior to almost all other approaches to ulcer healing, the levels of skill and training that are required, together with the need for frequent re-application of casts, have led investigators to search for simpler methods of providing the mechanical unloading that is necessary for healing to occur.

The key factor of a successful wound healing program is off-loading of the diabetic wound, as it is associated with reduced inflammatory and accelerated repair processes. Abnormal foot stress can be reduced using several different mechanical approaches, including callus debridement, prescription of special footwear, injection of liquid silicone, Achilles tendon lengthening, and so forth. Useful off-loading mechanisms include (1) reduction of walking speed, (2) alteration of foot rollover during gait, and (3) transfer of load from affected areas to other areas of the foot or the lower leg [110]. Plantar stress relief can be achieved using various off-loading modalities including accommodative dressing, walking splints, footwear, ankle-foot orthosis, total contact casts (TCCs) [111], post-operative shoes [112], cast walkers [28], and vacuum orthoses [113].

Footwear and orthotic devices also decrease strain of the plantar soft tissues. As pressure and strain are highly related, a small strain is associated with a small plantar pressure [114]. The most compelling evidence that off-loading accelerates ulcer healing comes from studies using a TCCs for healing non-infected neuropathic diabetic ulcers [111]. However, to optimize wound off-loading, the cast should provide total contact of the foot except for the wound site, which should be mechanically isolated [95]. The name "total contact cast" is somewhat of a misnomer. Almost all reported studies that have used TCCs to heal plantar ulcers have found typical mean healing times of approximately 6-8 weeks [14, 111]. Beside TCCs, the most useful prognostic feature of the healing time is the wound depth [109] and size [115]. Foot ulcers heal poorly if underlying tendons, ligament or joints are involved [109].

Armstrong and colleagues [18] found that the progression of ulcer healing using TCC, the mean duration of casting until healing was 38.8±21.3 days. The vacuum orthoses demonstrated a comparable pressure-relieving efficacy under the forefoot to post-operative shoes. Vacuum orthoses significantly benefit the redistribution of plantar pressure and the roll-over process during walking [113].

Conclusion

Diabetic foot ulcers result from abnormal mechanical loading of the foot, such as plantar pressure, pressure gradient, and shear stress. Prevention of diabetic foot ulceration is possible by early identification of the insensitive foot and by protecting the foot from abnormal biomechanical loading. The principles of good wound care include the use of proper footwear, use of appropriate antibiotics, debridement, control of serum glucose levels, and careful monitoring of the ulcers. There is clearly a need to further develop preventative measures on soft tissue biomechanics as well as improve treatment options to reduce the costs and morbidity associated with diabetic foot ulcers.

Acknowledgment

This study was supported by the Oklahoma Center for the Advancement of Science and Technology (OCAST HR09-048).

References

[1] NDIC, *National Diabetes Statistics 2011*, 2011, National Diabetes Information Clearinghouse (NDIC), NIH Publication No. 11-3892.
[2] WHO, Diabetes Mellitus, Report of a World Health Organization Study Group (Tech. Rep. Ser., no. 727), 1985: Geneva.
[3] Burns, S. and Y.K. Jan. Diabetic foot ulceration and amputation. In: Kin CT, ed. Rehabilitation Medicine. InTech Publisher, Croatia, 2012 (ISBN: 979-953-307-517-3).

[4] Palumbo, P.J. and L. Melton, *Chapter 17 Peripheral vascular disease and diabetes*, in *Diabetes in America*, U.S.G.P. Office, Editor 1995. p. 401-408.

[5] Reiber, G.E., E.J. Boyko, and D.G. Smith, *Chapter 18 Lower Extremity Foot Ulcers and Amputations in Diabetes*, in *Diabetes in America*, U.S.G.P. Office, Editor 1995. p. 409-428.

[6] Stockl, K., A. Vanderplas, E. Tafesse, and E. Chang. Costs of Lower-Extremity Ulcers Among Patients With Diabetes. *Diabetes Care.* 2004; 27(9): 2129-2134.

[7] ADA. Economic Costs of Diabetes in the U.S. in 2007. *Diabetes Care.* 2008; 31(3): 596-615.

[8] Saltzman, C.L. and D.A. Nawoczenski. Complexities of foot architecture as a base of support. *Journal of Orthopaedic and Sports Physical Therapy.* 1995; 21(6): 354-360.

[9] Cevera, J.J., L.L. Bolton, and M.D. Kerstein. Options for diabetic patients with chronic heel ulcers. *Journal of Diabetes and Its Complications.* 1997; 11(6): 358-366.

[10] Goodfield, M. and L. Millard. The skin in diabetes mellitus. *Diab tologia.* 1988; 31(8): 567-575.

[11] Reiber, G.E., L. Vileikyte, E.J. Boyko, M. del Aguila, D.G. Smith, L.A. Lavery, and A.J. Boulton. Causal pathways for incident lower-extremity ulcers in patients with diabetes from two settings. *Diabetes Care.* 1999; 22(1): 157-162.

[12] Pham, H., D.G. Armstrong, C. Harvey, L.B. Harkless, J.M. Giurini, and A. Veves. Screening techniques to identify people at high risk for diabetic foot ulceration: a prospective multicenter trial. *Diabetes Care.* 2000; 23(5): 606-611.

[13] Cavanagh, P.R., B.A. Lipsky, A.W. Bradbury, and G. Botek. Treatment for diabetic foot ulcers. *The Lancet.* 2005; 366(9498): 1725-1735.

[14] Sinacore, D.R. Total Contact Casting for Diabetic Neuropathic Ulcers. *Physical Therapy.* 1996; 76(3): 296-301.

[15] Caselli, A., H. Pham, J.M. Giurini, D.G. Armstrong, and A. Veves. The Forefoot-to-Rearfoot Plantar Pressure Ratio Is Increased in Severe Diabetic Neuropathy and Can Predict Foot Ulceration. *Diabetes Care.* 2002; 25(6): 1066-1071.

[16] Gefen, A., M. Megido-Ravid, M. Azariah, Y. Itzchak, and M. Arcan. Integration of plantar soft tissue stiffness measurements in routine MRI of the diabetic foot. *Clinical Biomechanics.* 2001; 16(10): 921-925.

[17] Klaesner, J.W., M.K. Hastings, D. Zou, C. Lewis, and M.J. Mueller. Plantar tissue stiffness in patients with diabetes mellitus and peripheral neuropathy. *Archives of Physical Medicine and Rehabilitation.* 2002; 83(12): 1796-801.

[18] Armstrong, D.G., L.A. Lavery, and T.R. Bushman. Peak foot pressures influence the healing time of diabetic foot ulcers treated with total contact casts. *Journal of Rehabilitation Research and Development.* 1998; 35(1): 1-5.

[19] Ledoux, W.R. and J.J. Blevins. The compressive material properties of the plantar soft tissue. *Journal of Biomechanics.* 2007; 40(13): 2975-2981.

[20] Cowley, M.S., E.J. Boyko, J.B. Shofer, J.H. Ahroni, and W.R. Ledoux. Foot ulcer risk and location in relation to prospective clinical assessment of foot shape and mobility among persons with diabetes. *Diabetes Research and Clinical Practice.* 2008; 82(2): 226-232.

[21] Oyibo, S.O., E.B. Jude, I. Tarawneh, H.C. Nguyen, L.B. Harkless, and A.J.M. Boulton. A Comparison of Two Diabetic Foot Ulcer Classification Systems. *Diabetes Care.* 2001; 24(1): 84-88.

[22] Treece, K.A., R.M. Macfarlane, N. Pound, F.L. Game, and W.J. Jeffcoate. Validation of a system of foot ulcer classification in diabetes mellitus. *Diabetic Medicine.* 2004; 21(9): 987-991.

[23] Schaper, N.C. Diabetic foot ulcer classification system for research purposes: a progress report on criteria for including patients in research studies. *Diabetes/metabolism research and reviews.* 2004; 20(S1): S90-S95.

[24] Lipsky, B.A., A.R. Berendt, H.G. Deery, J.M. Embil, W.S. Joseph, A.W. Karchmer, J.L. LeFrock, D.P. Lew, J.T. Mader, C. Norden, and J.S. Tan. Diagnosis and Treatment of Diabetic Foot Infections. *Clinical Infectious Diseases.* 2004; 39(7): 885-910.

[25] Robertson, D.D.M.P., M.J. Mueller, K.E. Smith, P.K. Commean, T.P. Pilgram, and J.E.M. Johnson. Structural changes in the forefoot of individuals with diabetes and a prior plantar ulcer. *Journal of Bone and* Joint Surgery - American Volume. 2002; 84-A(8): 1395-1404.

[26] Steed, D.L. Foundations of good ulcer care. *The American Journal of Surgery.* 1998; 176(2, Supplement 1): 20S-25S.

[27] Singh, N., D.G. Armstrong, and B.A. Lipsky. Preventing Foot Ulcers in Patients With Diabetes. *JAMA: The Journal of the American Medical Association.* 2005; 293(2): 217-228.

[28] van Schie, C.H.M. A Review of the Biomechanics of the Diabetic Foot. *The International Journal of Lower Extremity Wounds.* 2005; 4(3): 160-170.

[29] Arkkila, P.E.T. and J.-F. Gautier. Musculoskeletal disorders in diabetes mellitus: an update. *Best Practice and Research Clinical Rheumatology.* 2003; 17(6): 945-970.

[30] Dyck, P.J.M. and C.M.D.P. Giannini. Pathologic Alterations in the Diabetic Neuropathies of Humans: A Review. *Journal of Neuropathology and Experimental Neurology.* 1996; 55(12): 1181-1193.

[31] Caputo, G.M., P.R. Cavanagh, J.S. Ulbrecht, G.W. Gibbons, and A.W. Karchmer. Assessment and Management of Foot Disease in Patients with Diabetes. *New England Journal of Medicine.* 1994; 331(13): 854-860.

[32] Ledoux, W.R., J.B. Shofer, D.G. Smith, K. Sullivan, S.G. Hayes, M. Assal, and G.E. Reiber. Relationship between foot type, foot deformity, and ulcer occurrence in the high-risk diabetic foot. Journal of Rehabilitation Research and Development. 2005; *Journal of Rehabilitation Research and Development*(5): 665-72.

[33] Bus, S.A., M. Maas, L.A. de, R.P. Michels, and M. Levi. Elevated plantar pressures in neuropathic diabetic patients with claw/hammer toe deformity. *Journal of Biomechanics.* 2005; 38(9): 1918-1925.

[34] Boulton, A.J.M., R.P. Betts, C.I. Franks, P.G. Newrick, J.D. Ward, and T. Duckworth. Abnormalities of Foot Pressure in Early Diabetic Neuropathy. *Diabetic Medicine.* 1987; 4(3): 225-228.

[35] Bus, S.A., M. Maas, P.R. Cavanagh, R.P.J. Michels, and M. Levi. Plantar Fat-Pad Displacement in Neuropathic Diabetic Patients With Toe Deformity. *Diabetes Care.* 2004; 27(10): 2376-2381.

[36] Morag, E. and P.R. Cavanagh. Structural and functional predictors of regional peak pressures under the foot during walking. *Journal of Biomechanics.* 1999; 32(4): 359-370.

[37] Mueller, M.J., M. Hastings, P.K. Commean, K.E. Smith, T.K. Pilgram, D. Robertson, and J. Johnson. Forefoot structural predictors of plantar pressures during walking in people with diabetes and peripheral neuropathy. *Journal of Biomechanics.* 2003; 36(7): 1009-17.

[38] Ahroni, J.H., E.J. Boyko, and R.C. Forsberg. Clinical correlates of plantar pressure among diabetic veterans. *Diabetes Care.* 1999; 22(6): 965-972.

[39] Barbagallo, M., S. Novo, G. Licata, and L.M. Resnick. Diabetes, hypertension and atherosclerosis: pathophysiological role of intracellular ions. *International Angiology*. 1993; 12(4): 365-70.

[40] Lundbeak, K. Stiff Hands in Long-term Diabetes. *Acta Medica Scandinavica*. 1957; 158(6): 447-451.

[41] D'Ambrogi, E., L. Giurato, M.A. D'Agostino, C. Giacomozzi, V. Macellari, A. Caselli, and L. Uccioli. Contribution of Plantar Fascia to the Increased Forefoot Pressures in Diabetic Patients. *Diabetes Care*. 2003; 26(5): 1525-1529.

[42] Giacomozzi, C., E. D'Ambrogi, L. Uccioli, and V. Macellari. Does the thickening of Achilles tendon and plantar fascia contribute to the alteration of diabetic foot loading? *Clinical Biomechanics*. 2005; 20(5): 532-539.

[43] Katoulis, E.C., M. Ebdon-Parry, H. Lanshammar, L. Vileikyte, J. Kulkarni, and A.J.M. Boulton. Gait Abnormalities in Diabetic Neuropathy. *Diabetes Care*. 1997; 20(12): 1904-1907.

[44] Salsich, G.B., M.J. Mueller, and S.A. Sahrmann. Passive Ankle Stiffness in Subjects With Diabetes and Peripheral Neuropathy Versus an Age-Matched Comparison Group. *Physical Therapy*. 2000; 80(4): 352-362.

[45] Cavanagh, P.R., J.S. Ulbrecht, and G.M. Caputo. New developments in the biomechanics of the diabetic foot. *Diabetes/Metabolism Research and Reviews*. 2000; 16(S1): S6-S10.

[46] Sacco, I.C.N. and A.C. Amadio. Influence of the diabetic neuropathy on the behavior of electromyographic and sensorial responses in treadmill gait. *Clinical Biomechanics*. 2003; 18(5): 426-434.

[47] Sacco, I.C.N., A.N. Hamamoto, A.A. Gomes, A.N. Onodera, R.P. Hirata, and E.M. Hennig. Role of ankle mobility in foot rollover during gait in individuals with diabetic neuropathy. *Clinical Biomechanics*. 2009; 24(8): 687-692.

[48] Chao, C.Y.L., Y.-P. Zheng, and G.L.Y. Cheing. Epidermal Thickness and Biomechanical Properties of Plantar Tissues in Diabetic Foot. *Ultrasound in Medicine and Biology*. 2011; 37(7): 1029-1038.

[49] Hashmi, F., J. Malone-Lee, and E. Hounsell. Plantar skin in type II diabetes: an investigation of protein glycation and biomechanical properties of plantar epidermis. *European Journal of Dermatology*. 2006; 16(1): 23-32.

[50] Gefen, A. Plantar soft tissue loading under the medial metatarsals in the standing diabetic foot. *Medical Engineering and Physics*. 2003; 25(6): 491-499.

[51] Thomas, V.J., K.M. Patil, S. Radhakrishnan, V.B. Narayanamurthy, and R. Parivalavan. The Role of Skin Hardness, Thickness, and Sensory Loss on Standing Foot Power in the Development of Plantar Ulcers in Patients with Diabetes Mellitus—A Preliminary Study. *The International Journal of Lower Extremity Wounds*. 2003; 2(3): 132-139.

[52] Boulais, N. and L. Misery. The epidermis: a sensory tissue. *European Journal of Dermatology*. 2008; 18(2): 119-27.

[53] Zheng, Y.-P., Y.K. Choi, K. Wong, S. Chan, and A.F.-T. Mak. Biomechanical assessment of plantar foot tissue in diabetic patients using an ultrasound indentation system. *Ultrasound in Medicine and Biology*. 2000; 26(3): 451-6.

[54] Duffin, A.C., A. Lam, R. Kidd, A.K.F. Chan, and K.C. Donaghue. Ultrasonography of plantar soft tissues thickness in young people with diabetes. *Diabetic Medicine*. 2002; 19(12): 1009-1013.

[55] Hsu, C.-C., W.-C. Tsai, T.-Y. Hsiao, F.-Y. Tseng, Y.-W. Shau, C.-L. Wang, and S.-C. Lin. Diabetic effects on microchambers and macro-chambers tissue properties in human heel pads. *Clinical Biomechanics*. 2009; 24(8): 682-686.

[56] Cox, N.H., D. McCruden, A. McQueen, S.K. Jones, L. Ong-Tone, A.Y. Fixlay, and B.M. Frier. Histological findings in clinically normal skin of patients with insulin-dependent diabetes. *Clinical and Experimental Dermatology*. 1987; 12(4): 250-255.

[57] Reihsner, R. and E.J. Menzel. Two-dimensional stress-relaxation behavior of human skin as influenced by non-enzymatic glycation and the inhibitory agent aminoguanidine. *Journal of Biomechanics*. 1998; 31(11): 985-993.

[58] Kelly, S.B., J.E. Olerud, J.L. Witztum, L.K. Curtiss, A.M. Gown, and G.F. Odland. A Method for Localizing the Early Products of Nonenzymatic Glycosylation in Fixed Tissue. *Journal of Investigative Dermatology* 1989; 93(3): 327-331.

[59] Bailey, A.J., T.J. Sims, N.C. Avery, and C.A. Miles. Chemistry of collagen cross-links: glucose-mediated covalent cross-linking of type-IV collagen in lens capsules. *Biochemical Journal*. 1993; 296: 489-496.

[60] Menzel, E. and R. Reihsner. Alterations of biochemical and bio-mechanical properties of rat tail tendons caused by non-enzymatic glycation and their inhibition by dibasic amino acids arginine and lysine. *Diabetologia*. 1991; 34(1): 12-16.

[61] Andreassen, T.T., K. Seyer-Hansen, and A.J. Bailey. Thermal stability, mechanical properties and reducible cross-links of rat tail tendon in experimental diabetes. Biochimica et biophysica acta. *General subjects.* 1981; 677(2): 313-317.

[62] Brownlee, M., H. Vlassara, A. Kooney, P. Ulrich, and A. Cerami. Aminoguanidine prevents diabetes-induced arterial wall protein cross-linking. *Science.* 1986; 232(4758): 1629-1632.

[63] Oxlund, H. and T. Andreassen. Aminoguanidine treatment reduces the increase in collagen stability of rats with experimental diabetes mellitus. *Diabetologia.* 1992; 35(1): 19-25.

[64] Jørgensen, C.S., J.M. Ahrensberg, H. Gregersen, and A. Flyvberg. Tension-Strain Relations and Morphometry of Rat Small Intestine in Experimental Diabetes. *Digestive Diseases and Sciences.* 2001; 46(5): 960-967.

[65] Sun, J.-H., B.K. Cheng, Y.-P. Zheng, Y.-P. Huang, J.Y. Leung, and G.L. Cheing. Changes in the Thickness and Stiffness of Plantar Soft Tissues in People With Diabetic Peripheral Neuropathy. *Archives of Physical Medicine and Rehabilitation.* 2011; 92(9): 1484-1489.

[66] Gefen, A., M. Megido-Ravid, and Y. Itzchak. In vivo biomechanical behavior of the human heel pad during the stance phase of gait. *Journal of Biomechanics.* 2001; 34(12): 1661-1665.

[67] Hsu, T.-C., Y.-S. Lee, and Y.-W. Shau. Biomechanics of the heel pad for type 2 diabetic patients. *Clinical Biomechanics.* 2002; 17(4): 291-296.

[68] Caballero, A.E., S. Arora, R. Saouaf, S.C. Lim, P. Smakowski, J.Y. Park, G.L. King, F.W. LoGerfo, E.S. Horton, and A. Veves. Microvascular and macrovascular reactivity is reduced in subjects at risk for type 2 diabetes. *Diabetes.* 1999; 48(9): 1856-1862.

[69] Veves, A., C.M. Akbari, J. Primavera, V.M. Donaghue, D. Zacharoulis, J.S. Chrzan, U. DeGirolami, F.W. LoGerfo, and R. Freeman. Endothelial dysfunction and the expression of endothelial nitric oxide synthetase in diabetic neuropathy, vascular disease, and foot ulceration. *Diabetes.* 1998; 47(3): 457-463.

[70] Arora, S., F. Pomposelli, F.W. LoGerfo, and A. Veves. Cutaneous microcirculation in the neuropathic diabetic foot improves significantly but not completely after successful lower extremity revascularization. *Journal of Vascular Surgery.* 2002; 35(3): 501-505.

[71] Pham, H.T., L. Exelbert, A.C. Segal-Owens, and A. Veves. A prospective, randomized, controlled double-blind study of a moisturizer for xerosis of the feet in patients with diabetes. *Ostomy/Wound Management.* 2002; 48(5): 30-6.

[72] Schade, H. Untersuchungen zur organfunction des bindegewebes. *Ztschr Exper Path Therapis.* 1912; 11: 369-99.

[73] Zheng, Y.-P., Y.P. Huang, Y.P. Zhu, M. Wong, J.F. He, and Z.M. Huang. Development of a foot scanner for assessing the mechanical properties of plantar soft tissues under different bodyweight loading in standing. *Medical Engineering and Physics.* 2011(0).

[74] Horikawa, M., S. Ebihara, F. Sakai, and M. Akiyama. Non-invasive measurement method for hardness in muscular tissues. *Medical and Biological Engineering and Computing.* 1993; 31(6): 623-627.

[75] Zheng, Y.-P. and A.F.-T. Mak. An ultrasound indentation system for biomechanical properties assessment of soft tissues in-vivo. *IEEE Transactions on Biomedical Engineering.* 1996; 43(9): 912-8.

[76] Zheng, Y.-P., A.F.-T. Mak, and B. Lue. Objective assessment of limb tissue elasticity: development of a manual indentation procedure. *Journal of Rehabilitation Research and Development.* 1999; 36(2): 71-85.

[77] Ferguson-Pell, M., S. Hagisawa, and R.D. Masiello. A skin indentation system using a pneumatic bellows. *Journal of Rehabilitation Research and Development.* 1994; 31(1): 15-9.

[78] Vannah, W.M., D.M. Drvaric, J.A. Hastings, J.A. Stand, 3rd, and D.M. Harning. A method of residual limb stiffness distribution measurement. *Journal of Rehabilitation Research and Development.* 1999; 36(1): 1-7.

[79] Chao, C.Y.L., Y.-P. Zheng, Y.-P. Huang, and G.L.Y. Cheing. Biomechanical properties of the forefoot plantar soft tissue as measured by an optical coherence tomography-based air-jet indentation system and tissue ultrasound palpation system. *Clinical Biomechanics.* 2010; 25(6): 594-600.

[80] Kwan, R.L.-C., Y.-P. Zheng, and G.L.-Y. Cheing. The effect of aging on the biomechanical properties of plantar soft tissues. *Clinical Biomechanics.* 2010; 25(6): 601-605.

[81] Ling, H.-Y., P.-C. Choi, Y.-P. Zheng, and K.-T. Lau. Extraction of mechanical properties of foot plantar tissues using ultrasound indentation associated with genetic algorithm. *Journal of Materials Science: Materials in Medicine.* 2007; 18(8): 1579-1586.

[82] Pai, S. and W. Ledoux. The Quasi-Linear Viscoelastic Properties of Diabetic and Non-Diabetic Plantar Soft Tissue. *Annals of Biomedical Engineering*. 2011; 39(5): 1517-1527.

[83] Hayes, W.C., L.M. Keer, G. Herrmann, and L.F. Mockros. A mathematical analysis for indentation tests of articular cartilage. *Journal of Biomechanics*. 1972; 5(5): 541-51.

[84] Fung, Y.C., *Biomechanics: mechanical properties of living tissues*. 2nd ed1993, New York: Springer-Verlag. 568.

[85] Yarnitzky, G., Z. Yizhar, and A. Gefen. Real-time subject-specific monitoring of internal deformations and stresses in the soft tissues of the foot: A new approach in gait analysis. *Journal of Biomechanics*. 2006; 39(14): 2673-2689.

[86] Petre, M., A. Erdemir, and P.R. Cavanagh. An MRI-compatible foot-loading device for assessment of internal tissue deformation. *Journal of Biomechanics*. 2008; 41(2): 470-474.

[87] Patil, K., L. Braak, and A. Huson. Analysis of stresses in two-dimensional models of normal and neuropathic feet. *Medical and Biological Engineering and Computing*. 1996; 34(4): 280-284.

[88] Smith, K.E., P.K. Commean, M.J. Mueller, D.D. Robertson, T. Pilgram, and J. Johnson. Assessment of the diabetic foot using spiral computed tomography imaging and plantar pressure measurements: a technical report. *Journal of Rehabilitation Research and Development*. 2000; 37(1): 31-40.

[89] Gooding, G.A.W.M., R.M.D. Stess, P.M.D. Graf, K.M.D. Moss, K.S.B. Louie, and C.M.D.P. Grunfeld. Sonography of the Sole of the Foot: Evidence for Loss of Foot Pad Thickness in Diabetes and Its Relationship to Ulceration of the Foot. *Investigative Radiology*. 1986; 21(1): 45-48.

[90] Cavanagh, P.R. Plantar soft tissue thickness during ground contact in walking. *Journal of Biomechanics*. 1999; 32(6): 623-628.

[91] Erdemir, A., M.L. Viveiros, J.S. Ulbrecht, and P.R. Cavanagh. An inverse finite-element model of heel-pad indentation. *Journal of Biomechanics*. 2006; 39(7): 1279-1286.

[92] Zheng, Y.-P., A.F.-T. Mak, and A.K. Leung. State-of-the-art methods for geometric and biomechanical assessments of residual limbs: a review. *Journal of Rehabilitation Research and Development*. 2001; 38(5): 487-504.

[93] Veves, A., H.J. Murray, M.J. Young, and A.J. Boulton. The risk of foot ulceration in diabetic patients with high foot pressure: a prospective study. *Diabetologia.* 1992; 35(7): 660-3.

[94] Armstrong, D.G. and L.A. Lavery. Decreasing Foot Pressures While Implementing Topical Negative Pressure (Vacuum-Assisted Closure) Therapy. *The International Journal of Lower Extremity Wounds.* 2004; 3(1): 12-15.

[95] Petre, M., P. Tokar, D. Kostar, and P.R. Cavanagh. Revisiting the Total Contact Cast. *Diabetes Care.* 2005; 28(4): 929-930.

[96] Pitei, D.L., M. Lord, A. Foster, S. Wilson, P.J. Watkins, and M.E. Edmonds. Plantar pressures are elevated in the neuroischemic and the neuropathic diabetic foot. *Diabetes Care.* 1999; 22(12): 1966-1970.

[97] Mueller, M.J., D. Zou, and D.J. Lott. "Pressure Gradient" as an Indicator of Plantar Skin Injury. *Diabetes Care.* 2005; 28(12): 2908-2912.

[98] Zou, D., M.J. Mueller, and D.J. Lott. Effect of peak pressure and pressure gradient on subsurface shear stresses in the neuropathic foot. *Journal of Biomechanics.* 2007; 40(4): 883-890.

[99] Lott, D.J., D. Zou, and M.J. Mueller. Pressure gradient and subsurface shear stress on the neuropathic forefoot. *Clinical Biomechanics.* 2008; 23(3): 342-348.

[100] Lavery, L.A., D.G. Armstrong, R.P. Wunderlich, J. Tredwell, and A.J.M. Boulton. Predictive Value of Foot Pressure Assessment as Part of a Population-Based Diabetes Disease Management Program. *Diabetes Care.* 2003; 26(4): 1069-1073.

[101] Williams, R.B., D. Porter, V.C. Roberts, and J.F. Regan. Triaxial force transducer for investigating stresses at the stump/socket interface. *Med Biol.Eng Comput.* 1992; 30(1): 89-96.

[102] Lord, M. and R. Hosein. A study of in-shoe plantar shear in patients with diabetic neuropathy. *Clin.Biomech.(Bristol., Avon.).* 2000; 15(4): 278-283.

[103] Akhlaghi, F. and M.G. Pepper. In-shoe biaxial shear force measurement: the Kent shear system. *Med Biol.Eng Comput.* 1996; 34(4): 315-317.

[104] Yavuz, M., A. Tajaddini, G. Botek, and B.L. Davis. Temporal characteristics of plantar shear distribution: Relevance to diabetic patients. *Journal of Biomechanics.* 2008; 41(3): 556-559.

[105] Yavuz, M., A. Erdemir, G. Botek, G.B. Hirschman, L. Bardsley, and B.L. Davis. Peak Plantar Pressure and Shear Locations: Relevance to diabetic patients. *Diabetes Care.* 2007; 30(10): 2643-2645.

[106] Yavuz, M., G. Botek, and B.L. Davis. Plantar shear stress distributions: Comparing actual and predicted frictional forces at the foot-ground interface. *Journal of Biomechanics.* 2007; 40(13): 3045-3049.

[107] Stucke, S., D. McFarland, L. Goss, S. Fonov, G.R. McMillan, A. Tucker, N. Berme, H. Cenk Guler, C. Bigelow, and B.L. Davis. Spatial relationships between shearing stresses and pressure on the plantar skin surface during gait. *Journal of Biomechanics.* 2012; 45(3): 619-622.

[108] Cong, Y., J. Tak-Man Cheung, A.K.L. Leung, and M. Zhang. Effect of heel height on in-shoe localized triaxial stresses. *Journal of Biomechanics.* 2011; 44(12): 2267-2272.

[109] Leung, P.C. Diabetic foot ulcers—a comprehensive review. *The Surgeon.* 2007; 5(4): 219-231.

[110] van Deursen, R. Mechanical Loading and Off-Loading of the Plantar Surface of the Diabetic Foot. *Clinical Infectious Diseases.* 2004; 39(3): S87-S91.

[111] Mueller, M.J., J.E. Diamond, D.R. Sinacore, A. Delitto, V.P. Blair, D.A. Drury, and S.J. Rose. *Total Contact Casting in Treatment of Diabetic Plantar Ulcers: Controlled Clinical Trial. Diabetes Care.* 1989; 12(6): 384-388.

[112] Bus, S.A., R.W.M. van Deursen, R.V. Kanade, M. Wissink, E.A. Manning, J.G. van Baal, and K.G. Harding. Plantar pressure relief in the diabetic foot using forefoot offloading shoes. *Gait and Posture.* 2009; 29(4): 618-622.

[113] Nagel, A. and D. Rosenbaum. Vacuum cushioned removable cast walkers reduce foot loading in patients with diabetes mellitus. *Gait and Posture.* 2009; 30(1): 11-15.

[114] Lott, D.J., M.K. Hastings, P.K. Commean, K.E. Smith, and M.J. Mueller. Effect of footwear and orthotic devices on stress reduction and soft tissue strain of the neuropathic foot. *Clinical Biomechanics.* 2007; 22(3): 352-359.

[115] Zimny, S., H. Schatz, and M. Pfohl. Determinants and estimation of healing times in diabetic foot ulcers. *Journal of Diabetes and Its Complications.* 2002; 16(5): 327-332.

In: Soft Tissue
Editors: A. J. Chavez Ruiz et al.
ISBN 978-1-62257-363-9

Chapter II

Cellular and Physiological Soft Tissue Response in Hip Arthroplasty and Its Management

Shahril R. Shaarani[1], Tidi M. Hassan[2], Ann Igoe[2], Gavin McHugh[1], and Denis Collins[1]
[1]Department of Orthopaedics and Trauma Surgery, Beaumont Hospital, Dublin, Republic of Ireland
[2]Education and Research Centre, Royal College of Surgeons, Beaumont Hospital, Dublin, Republic of Ireland

Abstract

Metallic and non-metallic orthopaedic prostheses have been used widely to replace painful, stiff and mechanically disadvantaged hips. Though the biomaterials used in these implants have been generally considered as inert, adverse tissue reactions in metal-on-polyethylene and more recently metal-on-metal hip arthroplasties have been described since the early 1970s.

This can result in premature failure of these implants and need for revision surgery. Recently, a specific implant has been recalled internationally.

There has been a worldwide increase in the rate of revision surgery for hip resurfacing arthroplasty due to adverse soft tissue reactions. Inflammatory pseudotumours are a well-described clinical complication of metal-on-metal and recent evidence has suggested similar complications for non-metal-on-metal hip implants.

Metal hypersensitivity has been characterized by a predominantly lymphocytic immune response and causes soft-tissue changes such as effusions, pseudotumours and osteolysis. Radiological and histopathological studies have characterized this phenomenon with inflammation, with an emphasis on metal debris as integral to the pathogenesis of this phenomenon. Also, the carcinogenic properties of cadmium, chromium, cobalt, beryllium and other metals utilized in orthopaedic devices have been proven in animal models. This book chapter will discuss the biologic and physical effects of hip athroplasty on soft tissue including pseudotumours and hip arthroplasty-related malignancies.

Introduction

Over the last decade there has been a 32% increase in THA with approximately 153 per 100,000 population undergoing the procedure in 2008 [1]. This rise also correlates with the increase in life expectancy in EU countries by 3 years in males and 2 years in females. The increased rate of THA and the increase in life expectancy has brought concerns regarding implants to the fore. Metallic orthopaedic prostheses have been used widely to repair poorly functioning, severely painful and defective hips. Though the biomaterials used in these implants have been generally considered as inert, adverse tissue reactions in metal-on-metal (MoM) hip arthroplasty have been described since the early 1970s.

This can result in the early failure of these implants and a need for revision surgery.

Recently, the manufacturer recalled both the ASR XL Acetabular System and the ASR Hip Resurfacing System worldwide. There has been worldwide increase in the rate of revision surgery for MoM hip arthroplasty due to adverse soft tissue reactions.

This chapter will discuss the biologic and pathophysiologic effects of hip athroplasty on soft tissue and its management, an important health and economic issue in the area of current orthopaedics.

A Brief History of Biomaterials in Total Hip Arthroplasty

Orthopaedic implants are specifically designed devices that meet a particular function when implanted into an organic environment. The inorganic materials used in the industry are termed biomaterials, as they are intended to withstand and function within a biological milieu. A THA system with modular components can contain four or more different materials such as stainless steel, titanium, cobalt-chrome alloy, ceramic, polyethylene and polymethylmethylacrylate (PMMA or bone cement).

A hip prosthesis differs from static metal implants due to the liberation of metal and plastic particles from articulating surfaces that may affect the pseudocapsule, joint space and bone in a continuous fashion.

The earliest attempts of THA involved using various materials such as muscle, subcutaneous tissue, rubber, decalcified bone and pig bladder. These materials had unsatisfactory results [2,3].

In 1891 Germany, Themistocles Gluck produced an ivory ball and socket joint backed with nickel-plated fixation [4]. This was a fundamental success for future progression in THA design as Gluck's original surgical principles are currently being used today; stable fixation of the prosthesis, use of bone cement, modular component insertion and the concept of biocompatibility. Concurrently in the USA, Marius Smith-Petersen designed the first synthetic interpositional arthroplasty using a glass prosthesis [5].

This was prone to breakage and hence Vitallium, a cobalt chromium alloy, was later used with reproducible results. Various combinations of bearings in modular THA have been applied in the past. MoM THA were developed in the 1930s and developed further in 1950-60s by the pioneering work of McKee and Ring. Boutin used ceramic-on-ceramic (CoC) bearings in the 1970s.

During the same period, Sir John Charnley introduced the idea of low friction torque arthroplasty with the use of acrylic cement for component fixation [6]. His initial use of Teflon had high wear rates and it was not until 1962 that UHMWPE (ultra high molecular weight polyethylene) was popularized. The first generation arthroplasties had a 77% to 81% survivorship at 25-year follow-up [7,8].

1.1. The Human Body Response to Total Hip Arthroplasty

There are mechanical and biological factors that can promote initiate a series of events that leads to localized bone resorption and other soft-tissue adverse reactions post THA (Figure 1). Our chapter will focus on implant factors and the soft-tissue reactions such as osteolysis to foreign-body hip devices leading to pseudotumours and THA-related malignancies.

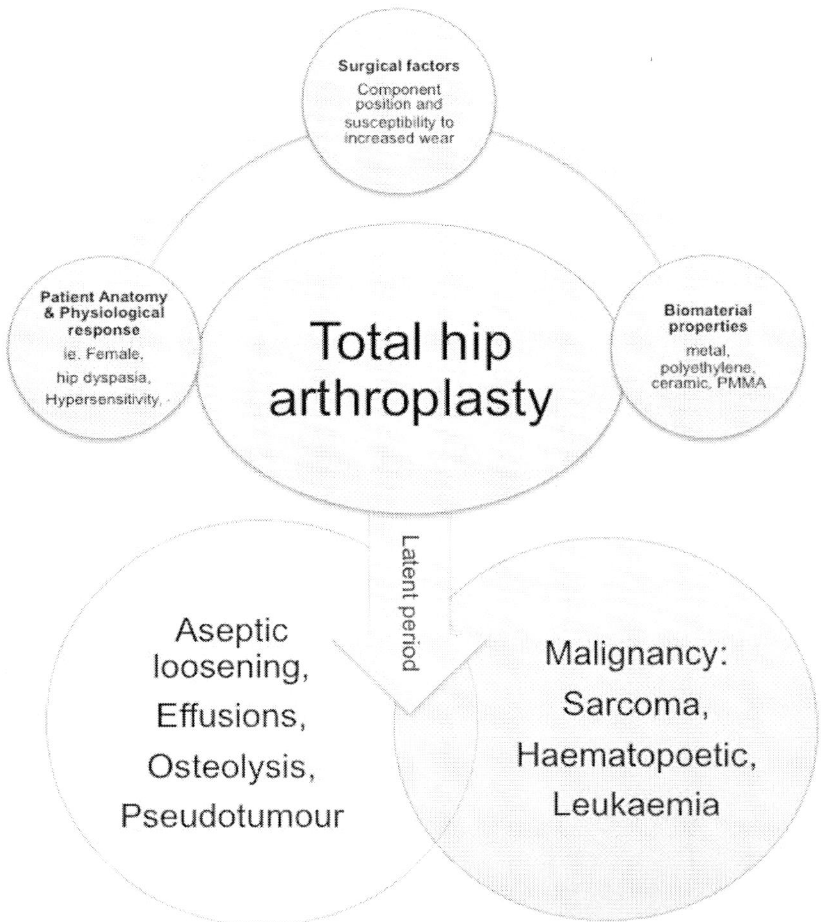

Figure 1. Flow diagram showing the factors involved in THA that increase debris wear particles, possibly leading to long-term complications.

Polyethylene Particle Disease

The particle disease theory was first described by Harris et al to explain the pathophyisiology of periprosthetic osteolysis (POL) [10]. Following activation by wear particles, macrophages and cells of mesenchymal origin secrete osteoclast-inducing agents such as cytokines, chemokines, and metalloproteinases [11]. This is coupled with a suppression of osteoblast activity by wear particles and cellular agents. Additionally, factors such as excessive force generation at the prosthesis-bone interface and intra-articular fluid production by the synovium macrophages further accelerate the enhancement of POL [12].

Frequent use of cemented THA such as the Charnley low friction torque hip arthroplasty brought POL to the attention of the orthopaedic community. Previously satisfied patients were presenting with insidious hip pain and follow-up radiographs revealed substantial bone lysis [9]. Erroneously termed "bone cement disease" in 1987, the phenomenon was eventually attributed to polyethylene debris. There are two distinct types of POL: linear and aggressive. Linear osteolysis is characterized by the formation of thin or heavy fibrous membrane deposition over sclerotic bone surfaces. Aggressive osteolysis is deficient of the sclerotic bone changes and instead consists of bony lesions filled with weak-supporting fibrous tissue. As a result of this misnomer, uncemented, biologic THA fixation was further researched and developed.

The rate of polyethylene bearing wear in THA is estimated between 1-5 x 10^5 micron-sized particles for each patient's step [13]. The debris particles are either phagocytosed directly by macrophages or after opsonisation by plasma proteins that trigger the release of matrix metalloproteinases, chemokines and cytokines [11]. This causes an increase in bone resorption by increasing vascular flow, recruitment of monocytes, activation of innate and adaptive immunity and reinforcement of multinucleated osteoclast formation and activation. Other cellular components like interface tissue fibroblasts (ITF) and osteoblasts have the same pro-inflammatory capability as macrophages. Larger debris particles require the formation of multinuclear foreign-body giant cells [14].

The main pathway in the mediation of osteoclast maturation and activation involves receptor activation of nuclear factor-κB (RANK) and RANK ligand (RANKL) [15]. Activation of RANK by its ligand leads to the activation of osteoclast-specific genes. Both TNF-α (tumour-necrosis factor-alpha) and IL-1 (interleukin-1) promote RANKL expression on marrow stromal cells, T-lymphocytes, ITF and osteoblasts and appear to be critical to osteoclast growth. Osteoprotegrin (OPG) however hinders osteoclast formation by binding to RANKL [16]. OPG is mainly secreted by dendritic cells, ITF, osteoblasts and their precursors [17]. Several studies have demonstrated the relationship between RANKL and OPG and the extent of the size on POL [18-20]. With the advent of polymerase chain reaction, the stimulation of gene expression of macrophages and other cellular components appears more multifaceted than previously believed [21,22].

Fundamental particle disease theory alone cannot explain differences in failure rates in patients receiving the same prosthesis and bearings [23,24]. Pokorný et al demonstrated that debris particles can reach a magnitude of 10^{12} with the average prosthesis wear rate of 0.1mm per year [25]. Several factors can explain the differences in the pathophysiology of POL. Hypersensitivity to prosthetic materials [26] and polymorphisms in genes encoding any of the mechanisms in POL (cytokines, hydrolytic enzymes, chemokines) can partially explain this reaction [27-29]. The coupling of endotoxins to debris particles markedly increases the physiological response to POL and it has been suggested that low-grade sepsis or systemic bacteraemia may be a causative agent [30].

The Metal Debris and Ions

Cobalt, chromium, molybdenum and nickel are all essential trace elements present in the normal diet. They are crucial for normal metabolic function and are detectable in blood and urine specimens of the general population. Cobalt is the metallic element of cyanocobalamin (vitamin B12) and is critical for normal brain function, nervous system and blood formation. Important cobalt-containing cofactors include methionyl aminopeptidase. Molybdenum is a vital cofactor for the enzyme sulphite oxidase which is essential in the metabolism of sulphur-containing compounds, hence important in the breakdown of toxins and hydroxylation of drugs. Chromium has a role in insulin and glucose metabolism. Chromium ions are present in two valencies, +3 and +6. Trivalent chromium is essential in normal physiological functions; however hexavalent chromium is a potential carcinogen. Excessive amounts of cobalt can cause goitre, cardiomyopathy, polycythaemia and cancer. These harmful effects are observations from animal studies and prolonged occupational exposure in humans [31-33].

The release of metal from joint replacements is the best documented form of internal metal exposure to result from surgical devices. This is due to the recognition of localized tissue response pathways to debris when implants were first introduced in the 1960s. Subsequently the success of joint replacement procedures has led to a significant amount of research into component design, materials and biological reactions that can possibly occur to improve the efficacy and longevity of the implants. Local tissue reactions from non-articulating surgical devices such as plate and screw fixations have lower debris levels compared to the joint replacement prosthesis.

Adverse tissue reactions in THA are best understood in MoM bearing surfaces due to the abundance of research material as well as the recent recall of a hip resurfacing system.

The first evidence of a local reaction to metal bearings was described by Evans et al in 1974 and was thought to be due to a hypersensitivity reaction to cobalt chromium alloy [34]. In-vivo metal sensitivity is characterized by predominantly lymphocytic immunological response and the pathognomic histological feature of aseptic lymphocytic vasculitis-associated lesions (ALVAL) in both the presence and absence of excessive metal wear [26,35,36]. Little consensus exists within the literature in defining the boundaries between ALVAL, metallosis and pseudotumours. However the former is useful in defining the histologic spectrum of arthroplasty failures associated with pain, a large sterile effusion and/or macroscopic necrosis or metallosis (Table 1).

MoM wear triggers the release of insoluble metal debris and soluble metal ions. High level concentration of prosthetic metal in the synovial fluid and capsule tissue has been reported both in fixed and loose prostheses [37-39]. The larger metal debris particles corrode and liberate further metal ions. The metal ions are absorbed into the circulation and increase the risk of a systemic build-up, but this is prevented by effective renal clearance [40]. The larger debris particles are phagocytosed or pinocytosed by macrophages and giant cells with intracellular chemicals (such as peroxides and chlorides). The lysosomes have the ability to degrade the debris into soluble metal ions (Figure 2). The lymphatic drainage is another clearance mechanism, where the metal particles are deposited in regional lymph nodes, liver and spleen [41]. Metal ions and engulfed metal particles can also induce cytotoxicity, chromosomal damage and oxidative stress.

Cytokines have a dual positive reinforcing and inhibitory role in the development of carcinogenesis. This system comprises of the macrophage-derived cytokines (TNF-α, IL-1, IL-6) and their interaction with eicosanoids (prostaglandin E2 and lipooxygenase metabolites) which control the expression of antitumour activity of macrophages from direct contact to tumour cells or from their cell-free soluble products [44].

Table 1. Histologic scoring criteria for ALVAL, a pathologic spectrum of an adverse reaction to metal debris in soft-tissue

Histologic scoring criteria for ALVAL score		
	Points	Characteristic
(i) Synovial Lining	0	Intact synovial lining
	1	Focal loss of synovial surface, fibrin attachment may occur
	2	Moderate to marked loss of synovial surface, fibrin attachement
	3	Complete loss of synovium, abundant attached fibrin and/or necrosis of lining fluid
(ii) Inflammatory infiltrate	0	Minimal inflammatory cell infiltrates
	1	Predominantly macrophages, occasional lymphocyte may occur
	2	Mix of macrophages and lymphocytes, either diffuse and/or small (<50% of hpf) perivascular infiltrates
	3	Mix of macrophages and lymphocytes, large (>50% hpf) perivascular aggregates may occur
	4	Predominantly lymphocytes, mostly in multiple, large (>50% hpf) perivascular aggregates, follicles may be present
(iii) Tissue organization	0	Normal tissue arrangement
	1	Mostly normal tissue arrangement, small area of synovial hyperplasia, focal necrosis may occur
	2	Marked loss of normal arrangement, appearance of distinct cellular and acellular zones, thick fibrous layer may occur
	3	Perivascular lymphocytic aggregates mostly located distally, thich acellular areas may occur
SUM		**Low= 0-4 ; Moderate = 5-8 ; High = 9-10**

ALVAL = aseptic lymphocytic vasculitis-associated lesion ; hpf = high-power field

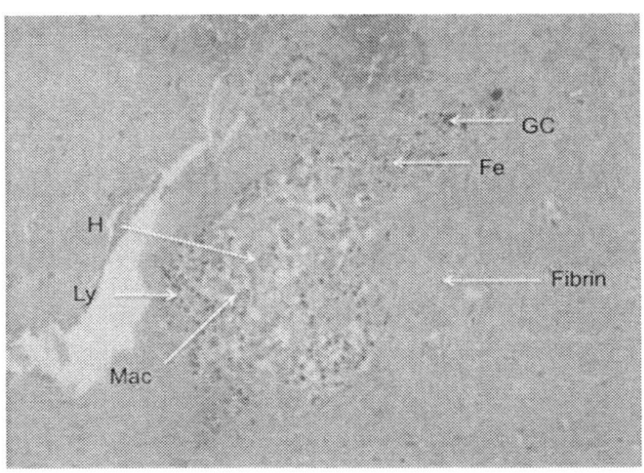

Figure 2. Microscopy slide displaying synovial tissue with macroscopic evidence of metallosis during a revision hip arthroplasty. There are underlying histiocyte (H), macrophage (Mac) and lymphocyte (Ly) cellular components together with a chronic inflammatory response. There are dark iron deposits (Fe) and multinucleated giant cells (GC) present.

Park et al demonstrated a higher incidence of hypersensitivity to cobalt ($p=0.03$) in patients with early osteolysis compared to controls [45]. The study had 169 THA patients with 2nd generation MoM prostheses, with 10 cases of osteolysis. Histological findings from 2 of the patients with osteolysis demonstrated perivascular accumulation of CD-3 positive T-cells and CD-68 positive macrophages.

Immunohistochemical studies have revealed the presence of bone-resorbing cytokines like IL-1B and TNF-α. This would suggest delayed hypersensitivity in MoM THA as a cause of early osteolysis. Milosev et al had similar findings with 591 MoM THA, where 25 cases had aseptic loosening [46]. Histological analysis in 17 of the cases demonstrated a hypersensitivity reaction in 13 patients (2% of total cohort), with perivascular infiltrate of lymphocytes and aseptic inflammation. One study demonstrated higher levels of serum IL-6 in patients who underwent THA after 10 years [47]. The serum IL-1β levels were also increased in patients with failing cemented titanium aluminium vanadium (TiAlV) prosthesis versus a control group [48]. These studies confirm that bone-resorbing cytokines are released into the systemic circulation in aseptic and sometimes loosening protheses and may prove useful markers for POL.

Ceramic Biomaterials

In non-metal-on metal (nMoM) bearings causing soft tissue reactions, the literature is more limited. Of 31 published case reports, the histological findings varied from cell populations of histiocytes, giant cells and foamy cells [49]. In the case of alumina ceramic-on-polyethylene and alumina ceramic-on-metal, the histological findings were similar to metal-on-polyethylene bearings [50].

Biomaterials and the Different Responses

The wear resistance of cobalt-chrome alloy is due to the inclusion of carbide (carbon) content within their configuration. These carbides can be depleted by the initial low-carbon form of the alloy or by the use of postcasting heat treatment during the manufacturing process [51-53]. The local consequences of wear debris are due to a combination of the total wear volume and the specific characteristics of the released particles such as size, number, shape, aspect ratio and bioreactivity. A study has demonstrated that the gravimetric rates in MoM bearings are more than two orders of magnitude higher than conventional bearings [54]. However this is offset by the fact that the size of particles is considerably smaller [55,56]. Particle sizes within the

0.2 to 7 μm are apt for phagocytosis. Metal particles are therefore more easily cleared, compared to polyethylene, due to its size and ion solubility.

There are differences between MoM and polyethylene debris leading to localized tissue clearance, immune activation and mechanisms and histopathology [57,58]. Polyethylene wear causes a preponderance of macrophages and foreign-body giant cell collection with birefringent polyethylene debris-filled histiocytes [59]. With MoM debris there are diffuse and perivascular infiltrates of T-lymphocytes and plasma cells, increased endothelial vascularity, fibrin exudation, necrosis and macrophages with inclusion bodies or metal particles [60]. These observations were first made by Willert et al which are a type IV delayed hypersensitivity response [61]. Metal-induced hypersensitivity is a delayed (Type IV) hypersensitivity reaction and is a cell-mediated response. This is in contrast to other types of hypersensitivity reactions, which are initiated by antibodies. The antigen binds to an antigen-presenting cell (APC) which is displayed with the major histocompatibility complex on its surface to be detectable to two kinds of T-cells: CD8 (cytotoxic) and CD4 (helper). The APCs also secrete IL-1 which further promote CD4 cell that secretes cytokines that mediates the immune response. Activated CD8 T-cells engulfs the target cells on first interaction, while activated macrophages generate hydrolytic enzymes and alters into multi-nucleated giant cells to further phagocytose the APC. This phenomenon may be related to ALVAL. POL and hypersensitivity are not analogous. Hypersensitivity is an abnormal immune response to all types of material debris causing adverse reaction to normal tissue.

The debate in the sequelae of particle disease is whether the body's physiological response is due to an innate hypersensitivity to metal or from an adaptive immune response due to increased wear. Caicedo et al [62] in 2009 have established a dose-related response to "Inflammasome Danger-Signalling Pathways" to cobalt alloy ions and particles [62]. Inflammasome is defined as an intracellular multiprotein complex that triggers the inflammatory response pathway including activation of IL-1β, TNF-α and NFκB that potentiates the inhibition of osteoblasts and maturation of osteoclast precursors leading to osteolysis.

This dose-related response suggests that painful MoM bearing failure is an expected response to excessive particle debris from sub-optimal functioning THA rather than a hypersensitivity response from a normal functioning THA [62,63]. Dorr et al argued that patients with undiagnosed pain with MoM THA are due to an increased generation of metal particulates due to excessive wear, rather than from a genetic predisposition for metal hypersensitivity [55].

1.2. Pseudotumours

A pseudotumour is a non-infective, non-neoplastic, granulomatous mass or destructive cystic lesion in close proximity to an arthroplasty prosthesis causing a localized complication. The exact cause of peudotumours is still not fully established. A common feature in recent studies has demonstrated increased wear due to either wear-prone bearing or from suboptimal prosthetic positioning. There is a variable time period of 2 to 15 years after the index THA before this foreign-body tissue response can be diagnosed clinically or radiologically [64].

Clinical Presentation of Pseudotumours

Pseudotumours often present with hip pain and discomfort, a palpable swelling or localized pressure effect from either MoM or nMoM THA [65]. A study in 1989 found that the initial clinical sign was stress pain, and further radiographic evaluation would exhibit a lesion around the THA stem [66]. Another study showed 65% of patients had discrete ovoid lucencies in or around the calcar, or the medial aspect of the stem. These lytic lesions are suggested to be precursor to pseudotumour formation [67].

MoM THA in particular have been associated with the production of cysts [68], solid [69] or semi-liquid masses [65] (Figure 3). The masses can exhibit an aggressive nature [65,70] and patients can present with a pathological fracture [71], spontaneous dislocation, and femoral nerve palsy [72].

Causes of Pseudotumours

The pathogenesis of pseudotumours is dependent on whether the causative agents are from polyethylene, ceramic or from metal causing different pathological reactions. The pathogenesis of pseudotumours was proposed to be multifactorial as an adverse event from overlapping soft-tissue reactions includeing metallosis, soft-tissue necrosis, allergy and hypersensitivity [71].

Several studies have investigated the cause of pseudotumours related to polyethylene wear. It has been described as an immune response to a foreign body to methylmethacrylate, polyethylene or metal adjacent to THA or total knee arthroplasty [64]. The debris is phagocytosed by macrophage giant cells leading to the secretion of prostaglandin E2, which creates a repetitive cyclical event of bone resorption and prosthesis loosening. Howie et al examined localized bursa formation in patients with metal-on-polyethylene hip resurfacings and ascertained the excessive wear of the polyethylene bearing as the direct cause of the mass [73].

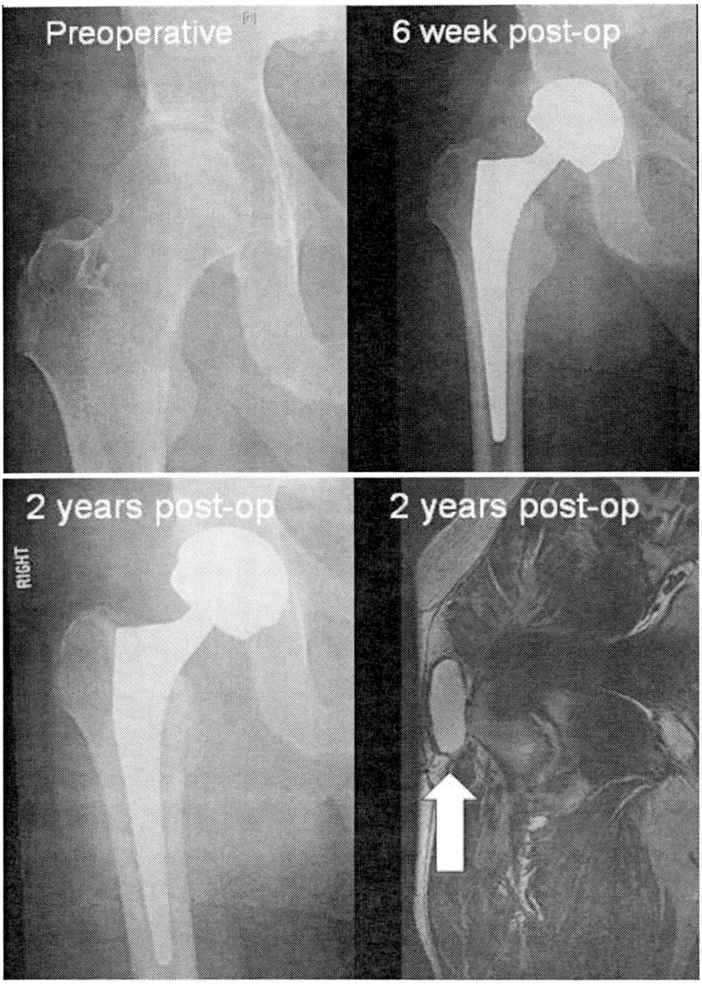

Figure 3. Radiological studies of a 55year old male who underwent a right stemmed MoM THA with radiographs taken preoperatively, at 6 weeks postoperatively and at 2 years post-operatively. Radiograph at 2 years post-operatively showed the prosthesis to be well-fixed. Magnetic resonance imaging, with metal subtraction, showed a large fluid collection on the lateral aspect of the greater trochanter (arrow).

Further studies have demonstrated polyethylene debris as the principal causative agent for granulomatous reactions [74-76]. It was also determined that UHMWPE as a single entity can generate a substantial osteolysis by producing foreign-body granulomas within the bone-cement interface [59].

A Danish study in 2006 examined 3 different THA bearing materials (zirconia-on-polytheylene, CoCr-on-CoCr and alumina-on-alumina) and established that granulomatous reaction is prevalent in well-fixed prosthesis even at 1 year post-operatively [77]. There was no difference in the macrophage and granuloma response to each bearing material. However since the metal and ceramic bearing were also seated within a UHMWPE liner, backside polyethylene wear could be a probable cause for the reactions. Another Scandinavian study demonstrated that destructive osteolysis also occurs in cementless THA and propose that granulomatous inflammation is not exclusively due to the biomaterial properties, but due to nonspecific foreign-body reactions [74,78].

In a study investigating revision of MoM THA, Willert et al analyzed periprosthetic tissue of 19 consecutive procedures [68]. Radiological studies preoperatively demonstrated radiolucent lines in 5 cases and osteolysis in a further 9 cases. Intra-operatively, both the acetabular and femoral component was well-fixed in 9 cases. The revision prosthesis was converted to non-MoM THA in 14 cases with the remainder 5 receiving another MoM-articulating THA. Interestingly, the latter patients had no decrease in their pain symptoms after revision surgery. Histological studies revealed widespread perivascular infiltration of T- and B-lymphocytes and plasma cells, increase in endothelial venules and fibrin exudation, a collection of macrophages with drop-like inclusions, as well as presences of eosinophilic granulocytes and necrosis. There was minimal metal debris discovered. This was an atypical type IV hypersensitivity reaction which caused ALVAL. However the study did not examine the primary THA components for wear pattern analysis.

Pandit et al discovered a necrotic granulomatous reaction similar in a delayed hypersensitivity reaction which may play a role in the formation of pseudotumours [79]. Metal debris particles were recovered in every case but there was only a weak correlation with component malpositioning, as the majority of their prosthesis was well-fixed and with acceptable acetabular cup inclination. However the anterversion of the cup was not analyzed. It was postulated that pseudotumours is partially due to the physiological response to increased debris accumulation from edge loading and also as a specific response of cobalt-chrome particles from the components. Further studies on the components revised in this cohort of pseudotumours were performed with the scientist blinded as to the indications for revision surgery ie. Pseudotumour, infection or fracture [80]. All the prosthesis revised for pseudotumours revealed evidence of edge loading proceeding to runaway wear. Interestingly, components with no evidence of edge loading had no pseudotumour formation.

Nolan et al demonstrated evidence of periprosthetic fluid-filled cavities together with widespread soft-tissue necrosis, tendon avulsions and proximal femoral diaphyseal necrosis, pathological fractures and dislocations [81]. This study correlated some or all the findings to the pitting corrosions evident on all of the femoral stems, even though these stems were well-fixed to the cement mantle.

Investigations into revisions of failed fourth-generation DePuy ASR™ cups in the Australian National Joint Registry implied that a reduced arc of cover progressed to an intensified failure rate secondary to increased debris production [82]. Other confounding factors were small-diameter bearings together with increased cup inclination and anterversion. The failure rate was 10.9% within the ASR resurfacings and 9.3% in ASR devices with femoral stems over a 5-year period.

McMinn et al also demonstrated that periprosthetic effusions are a consequence of increased wear from either edge loading or impingement [83]. This is from component malpositioning (i) from increased (>55°) or decreased (<35°) acetabular cup inclination, (ii) increased combined anteversion of the cup and femoral neck (>45°), (iii) or both. A suboptimal cup inclination in addition to an increased combined anteversion of the cup and femoral neck precedes to posterior impingement of the femoral neck at the edge of the acetabular cup and progress to increase wear.

These findings were more prevalent in females due to high incidence of undiagnosed hip dysplasia with associated torsional deformity in the younger cohort with early onset arthritis. Femoral anterversion in the range of 20-45° can be counterbalanced by reducing cup anterversion. Hip resurfacings are not recommended for femoral anterversion >45° unless performed together with a derotation subtrochanteric femoral osteotomy.

McMinn et al emphasized that component malposition cannot be excluded unless femoral neck anteversion is also analyzed. Malviya et al also postulated that edge wear and impingement to be the cause of pseudotumours [84]. All the above studies would indicate that the majority of periprosthetic-localized complications are due to component malposition in contrast to a native hypersensitivity response.

Further studies will require a two- or three-dimensional measurement of acetabular cup inclination as well as recognizing increased femoral neck anteversion preoperatively especially in the young female cohort due to higher incidence of undiagnosed hip dysplasia.

Management of Pseudotumours

Seventy-percent of MoM THR presenting with pseudotumours require revision surgery with a revision prosthesis combined with cancellous bone-grafting [71,85] (Figure 4).

The application of the revision arthroplasty should be appropriate for aseptic loosening. One-third of the patients will require subsequent surgery with a poorer outcome and functional score than after the index surgery [85].

Poorer outcome following surgery for pseudotumours could be related to the risk of recurrence which remains [86].

There is also a high rate of serious complications including recurrent dislocations, nerve palsies and femoral artery stenosis. Histologic ALVAL score should be used in all revision THA samples for standardized reporting [74].

Other masses in close proximity to THA that are malignant in nature, including soft and tissue bone sarcomas [81,87], lymphoma [87], and metastasis [88] are included in the differential diagnosis of pseudotumours.

Due to the presence of histiocytes, giant cells and necrosis, this reaction can also be mistaken with mycobacterial and fungal infections therefore must be out-ruled with acid-fast and fungal stains or culture sensitivities.

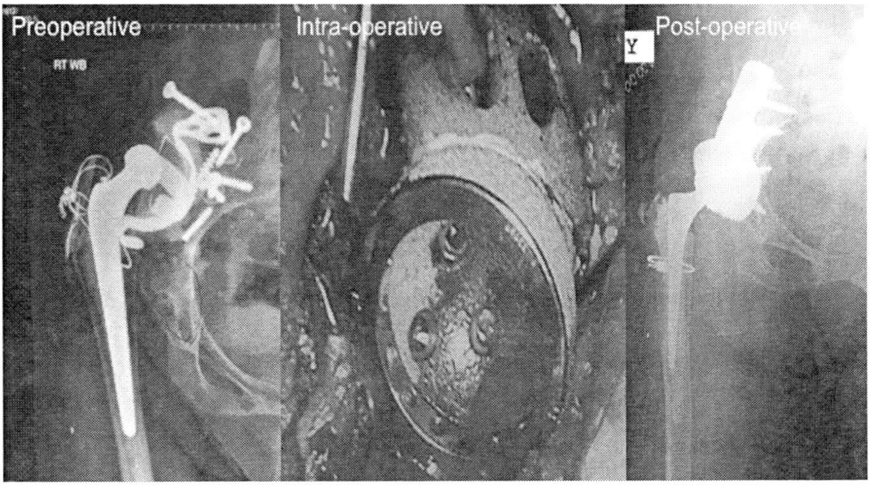

Figure 4. Preoperative radiograph of a failed revision arthroplasty with massive acetabular osteolysis and upward migration of the prosthesis. Intraoperatively the bony defect was filled with trabecular metal fixation, and exchange of the femoral stem. The postoperative radiograph shows restoration of the hip centre.

1.3. Malignancy Related to Total Hip Arthroplasty: A True Phenomenon?

Due to high failure of MoM hip replacement and the unknown biologic effects of metals, predominantly cobalt, chromium, and molybdenum, the risk of all type of cancers in post-THA patients have been speculated. After a hip replacement, metal particles disseminate throughout the body and can be found in blood, kidneys, liver, bladder and bone marrow [89, 90]. The pathway of internal debris or metal ions after a THA is shown in Figure 5.

A more recent and largest study in 2012 by Smith et al on behalf of the National Joint Registry in England and Wales analyzed 40,576 and 248,995 patients with MoM THA and alternative bearings respectively [91]. The adjusted five-year incidence of all cancers for men aged 60 was 4.8% with resurfacing, 6.2% with stemmed MoM and 6.7% for other bearing surfaces.

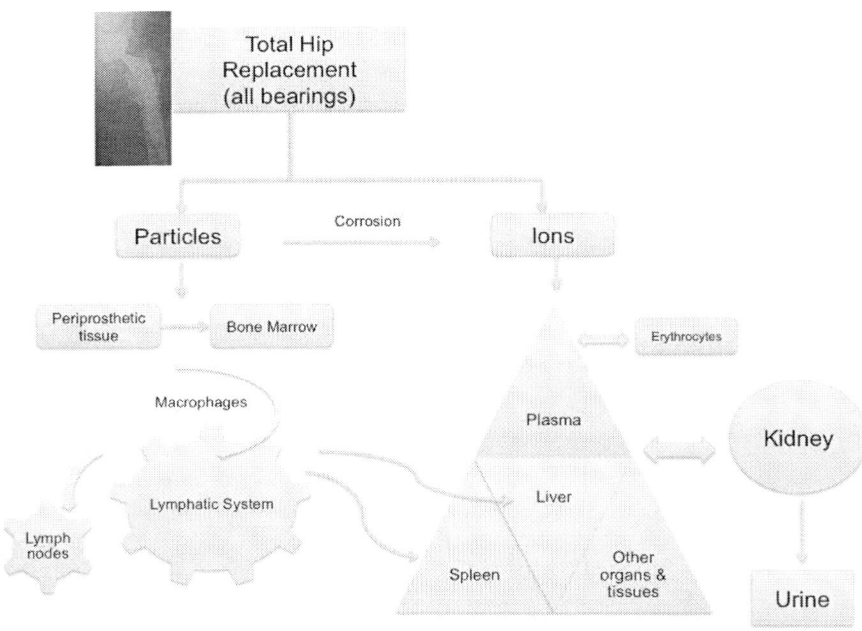

Figure 5. Internal exposure to particles and ions from a THA. Particles and ions released from the prosthesis can enter the systemic circulation where it can affect all organs with the eventual excretion from the kidneys. Debris accumulation within the periprosthetic tissue can incite localized pathologies, with macrophage phagocytic response and clearance into lymphatic system causing dissemination to distant organs.

There was no statistical significance between MoM THA and increased incidence of cancer. Interestingly, the cohorts who underwent resurfacing with MoM are less likely to develop prostate, haemotological or other cancers with a lower risk of death compared to the group who received alternative bearings. Data from Visuri et al for MoM prosthesis for specific cancers in his Scandinavian cohort revealed the relative risk of 1.59 for haematopoeitic cancer, 0.26 for sarcoma and 3.77 for leukaemia [87]. However the data was limited as the mean follow-up was 7.5 years and not adjusted for co-morbidities. Other epidemiological studies have also confirmed the low incidence of malignancy after THA, which have been pooled for a meta-analysis by Tharani et al [92]. The relative risk of all cancer for both MoM and nMoM was 0.97 with 1.02 for haematopoetic cancer and 1.03 for sarcoma. When the sub-group of MoM prosthesis was analyzed the relative risk for cancer was 0.95 whereas metal-on-polyethylene was 0.90. Although the incidence of malignant cancers in patients undergoing THA is lower than the general population, THA-related malignancies at the site of the procedure have been described. There have been approximately 50 reports of malignant cancers in patients after THA. The majority of cases were reported as malignant fibrous histiocytoma (MFH), a sarcoma mostly described as pleomorphic tumour with numerous giant cells.

To date, a review of 47 cases of malignancies at the site of THA was published comprising of 20 MFH, 9 osteosarcoma, 4 lymphoma, 2 fibrosarcoma, 2 leiomyosarcoma, 2 spindle cell sarcoma, 1 chondrosarcoma, 1 synovial sarcoma, 1 liposarcoma, 1 malignant epithelial epithelioma, 1 rhabdomyosarcoma, 1 malignant nerve sheath tumour, 1 giant cell and 1 epidermoid cancer [93].

Tharani et al reported a 2-year latent period in the development of malignant histiocytoma post-THA. For THA-related malignancies at the site of the hip replacement based on the 47 cases reported, the mean latent period was 6.0 years (range, 0.5–20 years) after the first THA [92]. Eighteen of the 47 tumors developed within 3 years after surgery. Cobalt-chromium (CoCr) and stainless steel were the most commonly used alloys. Older THA patients with articulating bearing surfaces, even without evidence of osteolysis or loosening of the implant have also been associated with soft-tissue sarcomas. More commonly, malignant tumours relating to the site of the THA are more prevalent in those with primary or secondary osteoarthritis as indications for the index THA.

Industrial and environmental exposures to Co and Cr are well documented [94-97]. In other medical fields, only chromium and nickel have been ascertained as a definitive cause of lung cancer in humans [98]. The carcinogenic properties of cobalt and nickel have been studied in animals. Intramuscular or intrathoracic injections of cobalt metal powder resulted in fibrosarcomas and rhabdomyosarcomas at the injection sites, while intra-tracheal infiltration of nickel metal powder produced lung squamous-cell carcinoma and adenocarcinoma [99]. Exposure to metal particles has recently been revaluated with the unearthing that nanometer-sized particles may be more toxic than larger particles. This concept of nanotoxicology is an emerging field and has become important in the orthopaedic community. The design of orthopaedic implants has changed over the last 15 years where there are an increased number of patients receiving hard-on-hard metal bearing with articulating surfaces comprising of CoCr. These implants generate mainly nanometer sized metal particles and ions. Prior to this introduction, majority of patients received a hard-on-soft bearing with the articulating metal of CoCr, stainless steel (SS) or titanium (Ti) rested on polyethylene. The implants produced mainly micrometer-sized particles and ions.

Literatures of Co and Cr exposures from surgical devices in human are limited and are fundamentally different from those induced by external sources. Since the contamination is derived from within the body, such exposures are different as these materials do not permeate across barrier membranes such as gastric or lung mucosa and skin. This is further termed as "internal exposure". In joint replacement prosthesis, Co (>34%) and Cr (>19%) form the combination alloy of CoCr used. Other metal such as nickel (Ni), molybdenum (Mo) and tungsten (W) were also used in combination to improve the physical properties CoCr. Cr also forms a percentage component of stainless steel.

The evidence for carcinogenic properties in implanted metallic components (chromium and titanium, cobalt- and titanium-based alloys, stainless steel) and organic polymeric materials are less established. Implanted metals of metallic cobalt, metallic nickel and alloy combinations containing 67% nickel, 13-16% chromium and 7% iron are however classified as possible carcinogens to humans [100]. Cobalt and chromium debris particles have induced carcinoma changes in animal studies [76]. Osteosarcomas and fibrosarcomas have also been found in cats and dogs with stainless-steel orthopaedic implants [102]. Interestingly, Lewis et al injected metallic alloy CoCrMo or TiAlV wear debris into knee joints of rats with no incidence of neoplasia on follow-up [103]. Current literature has mainly focused on MoM implant but there have been evidence to support the incidence of cancer associated with PMMA (bone cement) [101] and polyethylene [104] in animal studies. It is thought that the metal debris around the THA instigates a localized tissue response, which further propagates to mutagenesis [105].

The pathophysiology and association between neoplasia and the loosening of implantation of metallic components is yet unclear. The correlation of implant loosening and tumour in a rat study indicate that mutagenesis resulted from the reaction from the foreign body [106]. This relationship is not yet established in humans. Macrophages' attaching to implants result in the generation of reactive oxygen species (ROS) [107,108]. ROS can disrupt the host DNA causing mainly guanine-thymine transversion [109]. If these alterations are associated with oncogenes or tumour suppressor genes, then localized or systemic metal ion release can indirectly progress to malignancies.

Chronic inflammation is a precondition to malignancy [110] but this process has not been shown to be a causative factor as a result of prosthetic debris. The cytokine-related immune system could eradicate malignant cells around the THA in the initial phases. Further studies are required to investigate the effects of cytokines and particle-induced immune response in localized and non-localized tumours in THA patients. Other reported malignancies relating to the site of the THA could also be related to an occult or pre-operative tumour, in which the resected bone blocks at THA revealed cancerous cells pre-implantation.

Genotoxicity

Genotoxicity biomarkers have been considered to be prospective tools in relation to cancer risk in the future. Peripheral lymphocytes are often used to assess the incidence of genotoxic biomarkers exposed to humans due to easy availability. These markers include numerical and structural chromosomal aberrations. Numerical aberrations are depicted by a loss (hypoploid) or gain (hyperploid) of one or more chromosomes, which are termed aneugenic events. Structural chromosomal aberrations are divided into either chromosome-type aberrations (CSA) or chromatid-type (CTAs) aberrations. CSAs frequently involve balanced translocations and dicentric chromosomes whilst CTAs involve chromatid type breakages and exchanges [111].

Increased genotoxicity has been demonstrated in several studies with non-MoM and MoM THA [112]. In the absence of external factors in patient cohorts including smoking, there seems to be a relationship between implant and increased incidence of genotoxicity. Genotoxic biomarkers have been isolated in lymphocytes and buccal cells of patients with orthodontic devices, which imply that metal released from these implants have the ability to generate both local and systemic changes in cells [113,114]. Doherty et al showed an increase in non-specific translocations and aneuploidy in peripheral blood lymphocytes in patients with metal-on-polyethylene THA [115]. Patients implanted with titanium implants had a 5-fold increase risk of aneuploidy but no change in chromosomal translocations. Those with chromium implants had 2.5-fold increase in aneuploidy and 3.5-fold increase in chromosomal allocations. The same authors revealed both aneuploidy and CSA in patients with CoCr THA. However the prevalence of increased incidence of genotoxicity in metal implants was not significantly correlated with concentration of metal within the tissue specimen. Future studies are required to attain the relationship of genotoxic events occurring post-THA and risk of malignancy.

Total Hip Arthroplasty-Related Sarcomas

Malignant fibrous histiocytoma (MFH) is the commonest form of soft tissue sarcoma. Debris particles initiate an intense macrophage/histiocytic reaction, and the increased amount and activity of histiocytes possibly can increase the risk of carcinogenesis. The pathophysiology of MFH is yet unknown. Several cellular origins have been proposed: (1) fibroblastic (2) dual fibroblastic-histiocytic (3) primitive mesenchymal cells [116].

The first documented evidence of sarcoma in THA was in 1972 when a case of MFH was reported after 3.5 years following a McKee-Farrar THA [117]. From the approximately 20 cases reported in English literature, more than 70% of sarcomas occur in metal-on-polyethylene bearing systems, whilst 5 have been reported in MoM prothesis. These sarcomas were reported to be highly aggressive with complications including deep infection, chronic sinuses and Mafucci syndrome [87].

Bone infarcts are commonly associated with MFH [118,119]. Smooth surface, mature fibrosis, dormant macrophage activity, inflammatory reaction and close proximity of cancerous cells with foreign body such as metallic devices are potential precursors to mutagenesis [120]. Conversely macrophage response and porosity of foreign body surfaces for anti-mutagenic activities have inhibitory effects in sarcoma development [120]. Most studies have suggested that sarcomatous changes around hip prostheses are related to the wear particles of CoCr or polyethylene debris leading to toxicity and carcinogenesis. Two cases of MFH have also been described with an aluminum-oxide prothesis without evidence of osteolysis or prosthesis loosening despite the chemical stability and mechanical durability, as well as minimal debris due to low wear rates [121,122].

Kirkpatrick et al conducted an animal study with subcutaneous implantation of 15mm-disc of different materials: UHMWPE, PMMA, 99% purity titanium (Ti), nickel chromium, cobalt chromium alloy, and aluminium oxide (Al_2O_3) [123]. Localized sarcoma developed within 2 years in 12% of Ti implants and 35% in UHMWPE implants. There was no correlation between the different prosthetic materials and histology of tumour. Ti group had the highest rate of premalignant change with the lowest incidence of sarcomatous change. However these findings have not been correlated in a human study [124].

Total Hip Arthroplasty-Related Osteosarcoma

In the 9 cases of osteosarcoma relating to THA site, most were reported in the seventh decade [118]. Non-THA related osteosarcomas have a bimodal distribution with the majority of cases in juvenile patients and a second peak in the seventh/eight decade of life [125]. This second peak could be associated with Paget's disease, bone infarcts or radiotherapy. Small amounts of necrotic bone may remain after THA that could promote the occurrence of malignancy.

Bone infarction is associated with an increased incidence of osteosarcoma [126,127]. Animal studies have demonstrated the occurrence of osteosarcoma due to medullary infarction after THA and there is also a case report of osteosarcoma after a failed cemented THA in a dog [128].

This case reported a massive bone infarct distal to an uncemented femoral stem suspected 4 months post-operatively and further confirmed at 1 year. Polyethylene and CoCr wear particles were identified. Occlusive vascular fibrosis has been suggested as a potential source of bone infarction [129]. Although there are no case reports on the association of bone infarction and the occurrence of osteosarcoma in a post-THA individual, the pathogenesis between canine and human osteosarcomas are similar [130]. Therefore, we recommend close monitoring of patients with bone infarction subsequent to THA.

Management of Malignant Tumours Relating to Total Hip Arthroplasty-Site

The outcome for patients with THA-related malignancies has been poor with 77% of patients with sarcoma dying within 12 months of diagnosis. Treatment options include local excision, radiotherapy, chemotherapy, hemipelvectomy or femoral ex-articulation [81,121,131]. Wide femoral resection and/or prosthetic replacement with adjuvant radio- or chemotherapy are also an option. However, the choice of management depends on tumour size, local aggressiveness, systemic spread and grade of the tumour and any decision is made based on a multidisciplinary expertise including orthopaedic surgeons and the medical/radio-oncologists.

Conclusion

While THA has become a successful operation associated with excellent patient satisfaction, rare but serious soft tissue complications have been reported. From the limited published literature to date, these phenomena are speculated to be caused by a combination of foreign-body reaction, adaptive immune response including hypersensitivity, wear debris, aseptic loosening and possibly pre-THA patient factors such as gender, osteoarthritis and inherent risk for genotoxicity. The true prevalence of pseudotumours and THA-related malignancies is still debated. The low threshold for publishing cases of pseudotumours and malignant tumours at the site of the THA may in fact overestimate their importance. High quality cohort studies data from national joint registries with the help of diagnostic tools such as clinical, radiographic, pathologic, ion-level and genetic assessment will help improve our insight into these rare soft-tissue reactions in THA.

References

[1] *Health at a Glance: Europe 2010* - by OECD (Organisation for Economic Co-operation and Development, pg 97. Tables: http://dx.doi.org/10.1787/888932337129; http://dx.doi.org/10.1787/888932337167.

[2] Ollier L. Traité des Résections et des opérations conservatives qu'ont peut practiquere sur le sistême osseux. Paris, 1885. (In French).

[3] Chlumsky V. Zentralblatt für orthopaedische Chirurgie (Continued Centralblatt für orthopaedische Chirurgie un mechanik from 1887-1890). (In German).

[4] Rang M. Anthology of Orthopaedics. Edinburgh, London, New York: Churchill Livingstone, 1966.

[5] Smith-Petersen M. Evolution of mould arthroplasty of the hip joint. *J. Bone Joint. Surg. Br.*, 1948;30(B):59.

[6] Charnley J. The Man and the Hip. New York, NY: *Springer,* 1990.

[7] Berry DJ, Harmsen WS, Cabanela ME, Morrey BF. Twenty-fi ve-year survivorship of two thousand consecutive primary Charnley total hip replacements: factors affecting survivorship of acetabular and femoral components. *J. Bone Joint. Surg. Am.*, 2002;84A:171-7.

[8] Callaghan JJ, Albright JC, Goetz DD, Olejniczak JP, Johnston RC. Charnley total hip arthroplasty with cement: minimum twenty-fi ve-year follow-up. *J. Bone Joint. Surg. Am.*, 2000;82:487-97.

[9] Harris WH, Schiller AL, Scholler JM, Freiberg RA, Scott R.Extensive localized bone resorption in the femur following total hip replacement. *J. Bone Joint. Surg. Am.*, 1976;58:612-8.

[10] Harris WH. Osteolysis and particle disease in hip replacement. *Acta. Orthop. Scand.*, 1994; 65 : 113-123.

[11] Purdue PE, Koulouvaris P, Potter HG, Nestor BJ, Sculco TP. The cellular and molecular biology of periprosthetic osteolysis. *Clin. Orthop. Relat. Res.*, 2006; 454:251-61.

[12] Sundfeldt M, Carlsson LV, Johansson CB, Thomsen P, Gretzer C. Aseptic loosening, not only a question of wear: a review of different theories. *Acta. Orthop.*, 2006;77(2):177-97.

[13] McKellop HA, Campbell P, Park SH, Schmalzried TP, Grigoris P, Amstutz HC, Sarmiento A. The origin of submicron polyethylene wear debris in total hip arthroplasty. *Clin. Orthop. Relat. Res.*, 1995;311:3-20.

[14] Ma G, Ainola M, Liljeström M, Santavirta S, Poduval P, Zhao D, Chen T, Konttinen YT. Increased expression and processing of ADAM 12 (meltrin-alpha) in osteolysis associated with aseptic loosening of total hip replacement implants. *J. Rheumatol.*, 2005;32(10):1943-50.

[15] Boyle WJ, Simonet WS, Lacey DL. Osteoclast differentiation and activation. Nature, 2003;423(6937):337-42.

[16] Boyce BF, Li P, Yao Z, Zhang Q, Badell IR, Schwarz EM, O'Keefe RJ, Xing L. TNF-alpha and pathologic bone resorption. Keio. *J. Med.*, 2005 Sep;54(3):127-31.

[17] Koreny T, Tunyogi-Csapó M, Gál I, Vermes C, Jacobs JJ, Glant TT. The role of fibroblasts and fibroblast-derived factors in periprosthetic osteolysis. *Arthritis Rheum.* 2006 Oct;54(10):3221-32.

[18] Holding CA, Findlay DM, Stamenkov R, Neale SD, Lucas H, Dharmapatni AS, Callary SA, Shrestha KR, Atkins GJ, Howie DW, Haynes DR. The correlation of RANK, RANKL and TNFalpha expression with bone loss volume and polyethylene wear debris around hip implants. *Biomaterials,* 2006 Oct;27(30):5212-9.

[19] Mandelin J, Li TF, Liljeström M, Kroon ME, Hanemaaijer R, Santavirta S, Konttinen YT. Imbalance of RANKL/RANK/OPG system in interface tissue in loosening of total hip replacement. *J. Bone Joint. Surg. Br.*, 2003 Nov;85(8):1196-201.

[20] Veigl D, Niederlová J, Krystůfková O. Periprosthetic osteolysis and its association with RANKL expression. *Physiol. Res.*, 2007;56(4):455-62.

[21] Garrigues GE, Cho DR, Rubash HE, Goldring SR, Herndon JH, Shanbhag AS. Gene expression clustering using self-organizing maps: analysis of the macrophage response to particulate biomaterials. *Biomaterials,* 2005 Jun;26(16):2933-45.

[22] Guenther R, Morawietz L, Friederich M, Gehrke T, Frommelt L, Schröder JH, Krenn V. Expression of CD9, CD11b, CD18, CD52 and PDGFR-beta in the interface membrane of loose endoprostheses. *Pathol. Res. Pract.,* 2005;201(6):435-42.

[23] Gallo J, Havranek V, Cechova I, Zapletalova J. Influence of demographic, surgical and implant variables on wear rate and osteolysis in ABG I hip arthroplasty. *Biomed Pap Med Fac Univ Palacky Olomouc* Czech Repub. 2006 Jul;150(1):135-41.

[24] Wilkinson JM, Hamer AJ, Stockley I, Eastell R. Polyethylene wear rate and osteolysis: critical threshold versus continuous dose-response relationship. *J. Orthop. Res.,* 2005 May;23(3):520-5.

[25] Pokorný D, Slouf M, Horák Z, Jahoda D, Entlicher G, Eklová S, Sosna A. Method for assessment of distribution of UHMWPE wear particles in periprosthetic tissues in total hip arthroplasty]. *Acta. Chir. Orthop. Traumatol. Cech.,* 2006;73(4):243-50. Article in Czech.

[26] Willert HG, Buchhorn GH, Fayyazi A, Flury R, Windler M, Köster G, Lohmann CH.Metal-on-metal bearings and hypersensitivity in patients with artificial hip joints. A clinical and histomorphological study. *J. Bone Joint. Surg. Am.,* 2005;87(1):28-36.

[27] Malik MH, Bayat A, Jury F, Ollier WE, Kay PR. Genetic susceptibility to hip arthroplasty failure--association with the RANK/OPG pathway. *Int. Orthop.,* 2006;30(3):177-81.

[28] Savarino L, Avnet S, Greco M, Giunti A, Baldini N. Potential role of tartrate-resistant acid phosphatase 5b (TRACP 5b) as a surrogate marker of late loosening in patients with totalhip arthroplasty: a cohort study. *J. Orthop. Res.,* 2010 Jul;28(7):887-92.

[29] Wilkinson JM, Wilson AG, Stockley I, Scott IR, Macdonald DA, Hamer AJ, Duff GW, Eastell R. Variation in the TNF gene promoter and risk of osteolysis after total hip arthroplasty. *J. Bone Miner. Res.,* 2003; 18(11):1995-2001.

[30] Nalepka JL, Lee MJ, Kraay MJ, Marcus RE, Goldberg VM, Chen X, Greenfield EM. Lipopolysaccharide found in aseptic loosening of patients with inflammatory arthritis. *Clin. Orthop. Relat. Res.,* 2006;451:229-35.

[31] Grice HC, Goodman T, Munro IC, Wiberg GS, Morrison AB. Myocardial toxicity of cobalt in the rat. *Ann. NY Acad. Sci.,* 1969 Jan 31;156(1):189-94.

[32] IARC Monographs. Cobalt in Hard Metals and Cobalt Sulfate, Gallium Arsenide, Indium Phosphide and Vanadium Pentoxide. *IARC Monogr Eval. Carcinog. Risks Hum.,* 2006; 86.

[33] Excessive erythrocytosis, chronic mountain sickness, and serum cobalt levels. Jefferson JA, Escudero E, Hurtado ME, Pando J, Tapia R, Swenson ER, Prchal J, Schreiner GF, Schoene RB, Hurtado A, Johnson RJ. *Lancet,* 2002 Feb 2;359(9304):407-8.

[34] Evans E, Freeman M, Miller A, Vernon-Roberts B. Metal sensitivity as a cause of bone necrosis and loosening of the prosthesis in total joint replacement. *J. Bone Joint. Surg. Br.,* 1974;56(4):626.

[35] Jacobs J, Hallab N. Loosening and osteolysis associated with metal-on-metal bearings: a local effect of metal hypersensitivity? *J. Bone Joint. Surg. Am.,* 2006;88(6):1171.

[36] Watters T, Cardona D, Menon K, Vinson E, Bolognesi M, Dodd L. Aseptic Lymphocyte-Dominated Vasculitis- Associated Lesion. *Am. J. Clin. Pathol.,* 2010;134(6):886.

[37] Huo MH, Salvati EA, Lieberman JR, et al. Metallic debris in femoral endosteolysis in failed cemented total hip arthroplasties. *Clin. Orthop.,* 1992;276:157.

[38] Brien WW, Salvati EA, Betts F, et al. Metal levels in cemented total hip arthroplasty. *Clin. Orthop.,* 1992;226:66.

[39] Urban RM, Jacobs JJ, Gilbert JL, et al. Migration of corrosion products from modular hip prosthesis. *J. Bone Joint. Surg.,* 1994;76A:1345.

[40] Daniel J, Ziaee H, Pradhan C, Pynsent PB, McMinn DJ. Renal clearance of cobalt in relation to the use of metal-on-metal bearings in hip arthroplasty. *J. Bone Joint. Surg. Am.*, 2010;92(4):840-5.

[41] Urban RM, Jacobs JJ, Tomlinson MJ, Gavrilovic J, Black J, Peoc'h M. Dissemination of wear particles to the liver, spleen, and abdominal lymph nodes of patients with hip or knee replacement. *J. Bone Joint. Surg. Am.,* 2000;82(4):457–76.

[42] Lee SH, Brennan FR, Jacobs JJ, Urban RM, Ragasa DR, Glant TT. Human monocyte/macrophage response to cobalt-chromium corrosion product and titanium particles in patients with total joint replacements. *J. Orthop. Res.,* 1997;15(1):40-9.

[43] Nivbrant B, Karlsson K, K7rrholm J. Cytokine levels in synovial fluid from hips with well-functioning or loose prostheses. *J. Bone Joint. B.,* 1999;81B:163.

[44] Bonta IL, Ben-Efraim S. Involvement of inflammatory mediators in macrophage antitumor activity. *J. Leukoc. Biol.,* 1993;54:613.

[45] Park YS, Moon YW, Lim SJ, Yang JM, Ahn G, Choi YL. Early osteolysisfollowing second-generation metal-on-metal hip replacement. *J. Bone Joint. Surg. Am.,* 2005;87(7):1515-21.

[46] Milosev I, Trebse R, Kovac S, Cor A, Pisot V. Survivorship and retrieval analysis of Sikomet metal-on-metal total hip replacements at a mean of sevenyears. *J. Bone Joint. Surg. Am.,* 2006;88(6):1173-82.

[47] Hernigou P, Intrator L, Bahrami T, et al. Interleukin- 6 in the blood of patients with total hip arthroplasty without loosening. *Clin. Orthop.,* 1999;366:147.

[48] Granchi D, Verri E, Stera G, et al. Bone-resorbing cytokines in serum of patients with aseptic loosening of hip prosthesis. *J. Bone Joint. Surg.,* 1998;80B:912.

[49] Carli A, Reuven A, Zukor DJ, Antoniou J.Adverse soft-tissue reactions around non-metal-on-metal total hip arthroplasty - a systematic review of the literature. Bull NYU Hosp Jt Dis., 2011;69 Suppl 1:S47-51.

[50] Valentí J, Del Río J, Amillo S. Catastrophic wear in a metal-on-ceramic total hip arthroplasty. *J. Arthroplasty.,* 2007;22(6):920-2.

[51] Korovessis P, Petsinis G, Repanti M, Repantis T. Metallosis after contemporary metal-on-metal total hip arthroplasty. Five to nine-year follow-up. *J. Bone Joint. Surg. Am.,* 2006;88:1183–91.

[52] Milosev I, Trebse R, Kovac S, Cor A, Pisot V. Survivorship and retrieval analysis of Sikomet metal-on-metal total hip replacements at a mean of seven years.*J. Bone Joint. Surg. Am.,* 2006;88:1173–82.

[53] Daniel J, Pradhan C, Ziaee H, McMinn DJ. Ten-year results of a unique first-of-a-kind metal-metal bearing. *J. Bone Joint. Surg. Br.,* 2010; 92:20–7.

[54] Anissian HL, Stark A, Gustafson A, Good V, Clarke IC. Metal-on-metal bearing in hip prosthesis generates 100-fold less wear debris than metal-on-polyethylene. *Acta. Orthop. Scand.,* 1999;70(6):578–82.
[55] Dorr PF, Campbell PA, Worrall J, Benya PD, McKellop HA, Amstutz HC. Metal wear particle characterization from metal on metal total hip replacements: transmission electron microscopy study of periprosthetic tissues and isolated particles. *J. Biomed. Mater. Res.,* 1998;42(1): 103–11.
[56] Sieber HP, Rieker CB, Köttig P. Analysis of 118 second-generation metal-on-metal retrieved hip implants. *J. Bone Joint. Surg. Br.,* 1999;81(1):46–50.
[57] Endres S, Bartsch I, Stürz S, Kratz M, Wilke A. Polyethylene and cobalt-chromium molybdenium particles elicit a different immune response in vitro. *J. Mater. Sci. Mater. Med.,* 2008;19(3):1209–14.
[58] Willert H G, Buchhorn G H, Fayyazi A, Lohmann C H. Histopathological, changes in tissues surrounding metal/metal, joints - Signs of delayed type hypersensitivity? In: World, tribology forum in arthroplasty (eds. Rieker C, Onerholzer, S, Wyss U). Bern: *Hans. Huber. Verlag.,* 2001: 147–66.
[59] Willert HG, Semlitsch M. Reactions of the articular capsule to wear products of artificial joint prostheses. *J. Biomed. Mater. Res.,* 1977 Mar;11(2):157–64.
[60] Willert HG, Buchhorn GH, Göbel D, Köster G, Schaffner S, Schenk R, Semlitsch M. Wear behavior and histopathology of classic cemented metal on metal hip endoprostheses. *Clin. Orthop. Relat. Res.,* 1996;(329 Suppl):S160–86.
[61] Christiansen K, Holmes K, Zilko PJ. Metal sensitivity causing loosened joint prostheses. *Ann. Rheum. Dis.,* 1980;39(5):476–80.
[62] Caicedo MS, Desai R, McAllister K, Reddy A, Jacobs JJ, Hallab NJ. Soluble and particulate Co-Cr-Mo alloy implant metals activate the inflammasome danger signaling pathway in human macrophages: a novel mechanism for implant debris reactivity. *J. Orthop. Res.,* 2009;27(7):847–54.
[63] Shahrdar C, Campbell P, Mirra J, Dorr LD. Painful metal-on-metal total hip arthroplasty. *J. Arthroplasty.,* 2006;21(2):289–93.
[64] Griffiths HJ, Burke J, Bonfiglio TA. Granulomatous pseudotumors in total joint replacement. *Skeletal. Radiol.,* 1987;16(2):146–52.

[65] Counsell A, Heasley R, Arumilli B, Paul A. A groin mass caused by metal particle debris after hip resurfacing. *Acta. Orthop. Belg.,* 2008 Dec;74(6):870–4.

[66] Tallroth K, Eskola A, Santavirta S, Konttinen YT, Lindholm TS. Aggressive granulomatous lesions after hip arthroplasty. *J. Bone Joint. Surg. Br.,* 1989;71:571–575.

[67] Wirta J, Eskola A, Santavirta S, Tallroth K, Konttinen YT, Lindholm S. Revision of aggressive granulomatous lesions in hip arthroplasty. *J. Arthroplasty,* 1990;5(Suppl):S47–52.

[68] Willert HG, Bertram H, Buchhorn GH. Osteolysis in alloarthroplasty of the hip. The role of ultra-high molecular weight polyethylene wear particles. *Clin. Orthop. Relat. Res.,* 1990;258:95–107.

[69] Madan S, Jowett RL, Goodwin MI. Recurrent intrapelvic cyst complicating metal-on-metal cemented total hip arthroplasty. *Arch. Orthop. Trauma. Surg.,* 2000; 120: 508–10.

[70] Nolan JF, Darrah C, Donell ST, Wimhurst J, Toms A, Marshall T, Barker T, Case CP, Peters C, Tucker JK. Metal On Metal Hip Replacement. *J. Bone Joint. Surg. Br.,* 2008 vol. 90-B no. SUPP III 531-532.

[71] Pandit H, Glyn-Jones S, McLardy-Smith P, Gundle R, Whitwell D, Gibbons CL, Ostlere S, Athanasou N, Gill HS , Murray DW. Pseudotumors associated with metal-on-metal hip resurfacings. *J. Bone Joint. Surg. Br.,* 2008 Jul;90(7):847–51.

[72] Harvie P, Giele H, Fang C, Ansorge O, Ostlere S, Gibbons M, Whitwell D. The treatment of femoral neuropathy due to pseudotumor caused by metal-on-metal resurfacing arthroplasty. *Hip. Int.,* 2008 Oct-Dec;18 (4):313–20.

[73] Howie DW, Cain CM, Cornish BL. Pseudo-abscess of the psoas bursa in failed double-cup arthroplasty of the hip. *J. Bone Joint. Surg. Br.,* 1991;73(1):29–32.

[74] Santavirta S, Hoikka V, Eskola A, Konttinen YT, Paavilainen T, Tallroth K. Aggressive granulomatous lesions in cementless total hip arthroplasty. *J. Bone Joint. Surg. Br.,* 1990;72(6):980–984.

[75] Austin RT, Stoney PJ. Granulomatosis of bone from high density polyethylene. *Injury,* 1982;13(5):414–418.

[76] Santavirta S, Konttinen YT, Hoikka V, Eskola A. Immunopathological response to loose cementless acetabular components. *J. Bone. Joint. Surg. Br.,* 1991;73(1):38–42.

[77] Nygaard M, Elling F, Bastholm L, Soballe K, Borgwardt A. No difference in early cellular response of the pseudosynovial membrane after total hip arthroplasty: Comparison of 3 combinations of bearing materials. *Acta. Orthopaedica.*, 2006; 77(3):402–412.

[78] Lazennec JY. Unexpected bad mid-term results with second generation (Metasul) metal on metal THP 12 years follow up. Proceedings of the 15th Triennial Congress of Asia Pacific Orthopaedic Association. September 2007, Seoul Korea.

[79] Pandit H, Vlychou M, Whitwell D, Crook D, Luqmani R, Ostlere S, et al. Necrotic granulomatous pseudotumors in bilateral resurfacing hip arthoplasties: evidence for a type IV immune response. *Virchows Arch.*, 2008;453(5):529–534.

[80] Kwon YM, Glyn-Jones S, Simpson DJ, Kamali A, Counsell I, Mclardy-Smith P, Beard DJ, Gill HS, Murray DW. Increased Wear Of Metal-On-Metal Hip Resurfacing Implants Revised Due To Pseudotumors. Presentation # 664 at the AAOS Annual Meeting, New Orleans 2010.

[81] Keel SB, Iaffe KA, Petur Nielsen G, Rosenberg AE. Orthopaedic implant-related sarcoma: A study of twelve cases. *Mod. Pathol.*, 2001;14: 969-977. de Steiger RN, Hang JR, Miller LN, Graves SE, Davidson DC.

[82] Five-year results of the ASR XL Acetabular System and the ASR Hip Resurfacing System: an analysis from the Australian Orthopaedic Association National Joint Replacement Registry. *J. Bone Joint. Surg. Am,*. 2011;93(24):2287-93.

[83] McMinn D, Daniel J, Pradhan C, Ziaee H, Wingate J. 10-Year Results Of Modern Hip Resurfacing: Hip Function, Clinico- Radiological And Ct Scan Assessment, #P098 - American Academy of Orthopaedic Surgeons. Las Vegas 2009.

[84] Malviya A, Holland JP. Pseudotumours associated with metal-on-metal hip resurfacing: 10-year Newcastle experience. *Acta. Orthop. Belg.*, 2009 Aug;75(4):477–83.

[85] Grammatopolous G, Pandit H, Kwon YM, Gundle R, McLardy-Smith P, Beard DJ, Murray DW, Gill HS. Hip resurfacings revised for inflammatory pseudotumour have an poor outcome. *J. Bone Joint. Surg*, Br., 2009;91(8):1019-24.

[86] Maurer-Ertl W, Friesenbichler J, Liegl-Atzwanger B, Kuerzl G, Windhager R, Leithner A. Noninflammatory pseudotumor simulating venous thrombosis after metal-on-metal hip resurfacing. Orthopedics, 2011 Oct 5;34(10):e678-81. doi: 10.3928/01477447-20110826-32.

[87] Visuri T, Pulkkinen P, Paavolainen P. Malignant tumors at the site of total hip prosthesis. Analytic review of 46 cases. *J. Arthroplasty.*, 2006;21:311-23.

[88] Schmidt AH, V{alker G, Kyle RF, Thompson RC, Jr. Periprosthetic metastatic carcinoma. Pitfalls in the management of two cases initially diagnosed as osteolysis. *J. Arthroplasty.*, 1996;11:613-619.

[89] Dobbs HS, Minski MJ. Metal ion release after total hip replacement. Biomaterials, 1980 Oct;1(4):193-8.

[90] Urban RM, Tomlinson MJ, Hall DJ, Jacobs JJ. Accumulation in liver and spleen of metal particles generated at non-bearing surfaces in hip arthroplasty. J. Arthroplasty, 2004 Dec;19(8 Suppl 3):94-101.

[91] Smith AJ, Dieppe P, Porter M, Blom AW; on behalf of the National Joint Registry of England and Wales. Risk of cancer in first seven years after metal-on-metal hip replacement compared with other bearings and general population: linkage study between the National Joint Registry of England and Wales and hospital episode statistics. BMJ, 2012 Apr 3;344:e2383. doi: 10.1136/bmj.e2383.

[92] Tharani R, Dorey FJ, Schmalzried TP. The risk of cancer following total hip or knee arthroplasty. J. Bone Joint. Surg. Am., 2001 May;83-A(5):774-80.

[93] Tao K, Wang Q, Zhang XL. Aggressive giant cell tumor at proximal femur after total hip arthroplasty. Chin. Med. J., (Engl). 2008 Nov 5;121(21):2207-8.

[94] Lees P. Chromium and disease: Review of epidemiologic studies with particular reference to etiologic information provided by measures of exposure. Environ. *Health Perspect,* 1991;92:93–104.

[95] Lison D. Human toxicity of cobalt-containing dust and experimental studies on the mechanism of interstitial lung disease (hard metal disease). *Crit. Rev. Toxicol.,* 1996;26(6):585–616.

[96] Barceloux, D. Cobalt. *Clin. Toxicol.,* 1999a;37(2):201–216.

[97] Barceloux, D. Chromium. *Clin. Toxicol.,* 1999b;37(2):173–194.

[98] Peters S, Vermeulen R, Olsson A, Van Gelder R, Kendzia B, Vincent R, et al. Development of an exposure measurement database on five lung carcinogens (ExpoSYN) for quantitative retrospective occupational exposure assessment. Ann. Occup. Hyg., 2012 Jan;56(1):70-9.

[99] McGregor DB, Baan RA, Partensky C, Rice JM, Wilbourn JD. Evaluation of the carcinogenic risks to humans associated with surgical implants and other foreign bodies - a report of an IARC Monographs Programme Meeting. International Agency for Research on Cancer. *Eur. J. Cancer,* 2000;36(3):307-13.

[100] Composite medical and dental implants. IARC monographs on the evaluation of carcinogenic risks to humans. Surgical implants and other foreign bodies, vol. 74. Lyon (France): *IARC;* 1999. p. 132.

[101] Heath JC, Freeman MA, Swanson SA. Carcinogenic properties of wear particles from prostheses made in cobalt-chromium alloy. *Lancet,* 1971;1:564-6.

[102] Black J. Orthopedic Biomaterials in Research and Practice. New York: Churchill Livingstone; 1988.

[103] Lewis CG, Belniak RM, Plowman MC, Hopfer SM, Knight JA, Sunderman FW, Jr. Intraarticular carcinogenesis bioassays of CoCrMo and TiAlV alloys in rats. *J. Arthroplasty,* 1995;10(1):75-82.

[104] Memoli VA, Urban RM, Alroy J, Galante JO. Malignant neoplasms associated with orthopedic implant materials in rats. *J. Orthop. Res.,* 1986;4:346-55.

[105] Swanson SA, Freeman MA, Heath JC. Laboratory tests on total hip joint replacement prosthesis. *J. Bone Joint. Surg. Am.,* 1973;55:759e73.

[106] Bouchard PR, Black J, Albrecht BA, Kaderly RE, Galante JO, Pauli BU. Carcinogenicity of CoCrMo (F-75) implants in the rat. *J. Biomed. Mater. Res.,* 1996;32(1):37-44.

[107] Adams DO, Hamilton TA. The cell biology of macrophage activation. *Annu. Rev. Immunol.,* 1984;2:283-318.

[108] Cross AR, Jones OT. Enzymic mechanisms of superoxide production. *Biochim. Biophys. Acta.,* 1991;1057(3):281-98.

[109] Waris G, Ahsan H. Reactive oxygen species: role in the development of cancer and various chronic conditions. *J. Carcinog.,* 2006;5:14. O'Byrne KJ, Dalgleish AG. Chronic immune activation and inflammation as the cause of malignancy. *Br. J. Cancer,* 2001;85:473.

[110] Mateuca, R., Lombaert, N. et al. (2006). Chromosomal changes: induction, detection methods and applicability in human biomonitoring. *Biochimie,* 88(11):1515–1531.

[111] Keegan GM, Learmonth ID, Case CP. A systematic comparison of the actual, potential, and theoretical health effects of cobalt and chromium exposures from industry and surgical implants. Crit. Rev. Toxicol., 2008;38(8):645-74.

[112] Burgaz, S., Demircigil, G, Yilmazer M, Ertaş N, Kemaloglu Y, Burgaz Y. Assessment of cytogenetic damage in lymphocytes and in exfoliated nasal cells of dental laboratory technicians exposed to chromium, cobalt, and nickel. *Mutat. Res.,* 2002;521(1–2):47–56.

[113] Faccioni, F., Franceschetti, P. Cerpelloni M, Fracasso ME. In vivo study on metal release from fixed orthodontic appliances and DNA damage in oral mucosa cells. *Am. J. Orthod. Dentofacial Orthop.,* 2003;124 (6):687–693; discussion, 693–694.

[114] Doherty AT, Howell RT, Ellis LA, Bisbinas I, Learmonth ID, Newson R, Case CP. Increased chromosome translocations and aneuploidy in peripheral blood lymphocytes of patients having revision arthroplasty of the hip. *J. Bone Joint. Surg. Br.,* 2001;83(7):1075–81.

[115] Fletcher C, Gustafson P, Rydholm A, Willén H, Akerman M. Clinicopathologic re-evaluation of 100 malignant fibrous histiocytomas: prognostic relevance of subclassification. *J. Clin. Oncol.,* 2001;19:3045.

[116] Swann M. Malignant soft-tissue tumour at the site of a total hip replacement. *J. Bone Joint. Surg. Br.,* 1984;66:629-31.

[117] Desai P, Perino G, Present D, Steiner GC. Sarcoma in association with bone infarcts. Report of five cases. *Arch. Pathol. Lab. Med.,* 1996 May;120(5):482-9.

[118] Bahk WJ, Lee AH, Kang YK, Park JM, Chung YG, Shin DS, Choi JH.

[119] Infarct associated sarcoma: a possible pathogenesis based on histological observation of repair tissue origin in two cases. *Acta. Oncol.,* 2010 Aug;49(6):868-72.

[120] Brand KG. Do implanted medical devices cause cancer? *J. Biomater. Appl.,* 1994;8:325.

[121] Ryu RK, Bovill Jr EG, Skinner HB, et al. Soft tissue sarcoma associated with aluminum oxide ceramic total hip arthroplasty. A case report. *Clin. Orthop. Relat. Res.,* 1987 Mar;(216):207-12.

[122] Yoon PW, Jang WY, Yoo JJ, Yoon KS, Kim HJ. Malignant fibrous histiocytoma at the site of an alumina-on-alumina-bearing total hip arthroplasty mimicking infected trochanteric bursitis. *J. Arthroplasty.,* 2012 Feb;27(2):324.e9-324.e12.

[123] Kirkpatrick CJ, Alves A, Köhler H, Kriegsmann J, Bittinger F, Otto M, Williams DF, Eloy R. Biomaterial-induced sarcoma: A novel model to study preneoplastic change. *Am. J. Pathol.,* 2000 Apr;156(4):1455-67.
[124] Brand KG, Brand I. Risk assessment of carcinogenesis at implantation sites. *Plast. Reconstr. Surg.,* 1980;66:591.
[125] Grimer RJ, Cannon SR, Taminiau AM, et al. Osteosarcoma over age of forty. *Eur. J. Cancer,* 2003;39:157.
[126] Galli SJ, Weintraub HP, Proppe KH: Malignant fibrous histiocytoma and pleomorphic sarcoma in association with medullary bone infarcts. *Cancer,* 1978;41:607-619.
[127] Sanerkin NG, Woods CG: Fibrosarcomas and malignant fibrous histiocytomata arising in relation to enchondromata. *J. Bone Joint. Surg. Br.,* 1979;61:366-372.
[128] Roe SC, De Young D, Weinstock D, Kyles A. Osteosarcoma eight years after total hip arthroplasty. *Vet. Surg.,* 1996; 25:70-74.
[129] Dubelzig RR, Biery DN, Brodey RS. Bone sarcomas associated with multifocal medullary bone infarction in dogs. *J. Am. Vet. Med. Assoc.,* 1981;179:64-68. 18.
[130] Withrow SJ, Powers BE, Straw RC, Wilkins RM.Comparative aspects of osteosarcoma: dog versus man. *Clin. Orthop.,* 1991;270:159-168.
[131] Syed AA, Agarwal M, Fenelon G, Toner M. Osseous malignant non–Hodgkin's lymphoma associated with total hip replacement. *Leuk. Lymphoma,* 2002;43:2213.

In: Soft Tissue
Editors: A. J. Chavez Ruiz et al.
ISBN 978-1-62257-363-9

Chapter III

A Histologic Study of Peri-Implant Soft Tissues: Orthodontic's Anchorage Miniscrews

***Farid Bourzgui*[1], *Mourad Sebbar*[1], *Samir Diouny*[2], *Zakaria Bentahar*[1], *and Farid El Quars*[1]**
[1]Department of Dento-facial Orthopedic, Faculty of Dental Medicine, Hassan II Ain Chok University in Casablanca, Morocco
[2]Chouaib Doukkali University, El-Jadida, Morocco

Abstract

For the orthodontist, orthodontic anchorage has always been a challenge because of tooth movement under the influence of forces applied to them. The use of conventional anchorage (elastic and removable extraoral face-bow) has certain drawbacks for the practitioner and the patient, including full cooperation on the part of that, some degree of discomfort and undesirable side effects [1]. The minimplant can be used for both horizontal and vertical orthodontic traction; they are small enough to fit between the mesial and distal roots of the molars for their intrusion. Placed in the palatal area, these miniscrews can produce sufficient anchorage for molar distalization. Note that miniscrews are too small to cause irreversible bone damage. They can be submitted at any time when the orthodontist or the patient wants and bone healing after removal is done without any incident [2, 3]. These anchoring devices have successes but also failures with particular problems of soft tissue inflammation, problems with patient comfort, the difficulties associated with the development of mechanics and orthodontic appliance on them (springs, chains...), stability problems of anchoring device, and removal [4]. Experimental studies, especially on the animal model, were able to study the various functional and morphological responses of both implants used for orthodontic anchorage (surface geometry), as the surrounding tissue (especially bone surrounding the implant). Various studies have investigated the histological, histo-morphometric and microscopic bone-implant interface [5,6,7,8,9,10]. However, the different reactions of the peri-implant tissues, especially soft tissue, are not yet widely studied. Little information is available on the influence of miniscrew on the development and maintenance of the barrier of peri-implant soft tissues. Current knowledge about the barrier of soft tissue is based primarily on animal experiments. However, the results of animal studies do not always correspond to the biological behavior of soft tissue in humans. For practical and ethical reasons, the study in humans is usually subject to differences in the parameters influencing the tissue response such as changes in local conditions of the mucosa, healing time, patient age, smoking and others.

In addition, these orthodontics' devices in oral environment are subject to electrochemical corrosion [11]; they may not only generate a progressive biodegradation of the material on the surface, but also of the oxidation process to release potentially allergenic and harmful substances. It is important to note that surface mini-screws tribological properties in orthodontics have been poorly investigated; in addition, their complex approach represent a major "challenge" for orthodontists.

This chapter aims to highlight the influence of the oral and orthodontic load on surface properties of mini-screws. It focuses on the prevalence of use of mini-screws in accordance with clinical indications, location and duration of active treatment; furthermore, in this chapter, we will investigate the different histological reactions of peri-implant soft tissues and changes affecting the state of surface miniscrews collected after orthodontic treatment.

1. Introduction

Orthodontic anchorage has always been a difficult and unpredictable challenge for orthodontists; this condition results when tooth movement is under the influence of force application. It has been documented that the use of conventional anchorage (elastic and removable extra- oral face-bow) has certain drawbacks (i.e. some degree of discomfort and undesirable side effects) for both practitioners and patients; it also requires full cooperation from the patients (Riendeau, 2003).

Miniscrews can be used for both horizontal and vertical orthodontic traction; they are small enough to fit between the mesial and distal roots of the molars for their intrusion. Placed in the palatal area, these miniscrews can produce sufficient anchorage for molar distalization (Figures 1.2.3). It is important to note that miniscrews are too small to cause irreversible bone damage. They can be submitted at any time when the orthodontist or the patient wants and bone healing after removal is done without any incident (Massif et al., 2006; Davarpanah et al., 2007).

These anchoring devices have shown success, but have also demonstrated failure with a particular reference to soft tissue inflammation, patient comfort, mechanics development difficulties and orthodontic appliance on them (springs, chains...), stability problems of anchoring device, and removal (Philippart et al., 2004; Buchter et al., 2006).

A various functional and morphological responses of both miniscrews used for orthodontic anchorage (surface geometry), as the surrounding tissue (especially bone surrounding the implant). More recently, however, several researchers have investigated the histological, histo-morphometric and microscopic bone-implant interface (Cornelis et al., 2007; Melsen et al. 2000; Buchter et al., 2006; Kim et al., 2005; Oyonarte et al., 2005). However, the different reactions of the peri-implant tissues, especially soft tissues, have been poorly studied. Little research is available on the influence of mini-screws on the development and maintenance of the barrier of peri-implant soft tissues. Current literature with regard to soft tissue barrier is primarily based on animal experiments. However, the results of animal studies do not always correspond to the biological behavior of soft tissues in humans.

For practical and ethical reasons, the study in humans is usually subject to differences in terms of the parameters influencing the tissue response; these include changes in local conditions of the mucosa, healing time, the age of patient, smoking, etc.

In addition, these orthodontic oral environment devices are subject to electrochemical corrosion (Naim et al., 1998), which may not only generate a progressive biodegradation of the material on the surface, but also of the oxidation process to release potentially harmful and allergic substances.

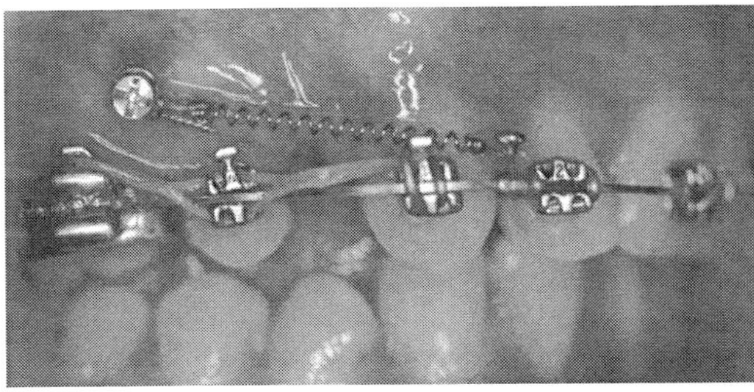

Figure 1. Mass retraction with orthodontics mini-screws.

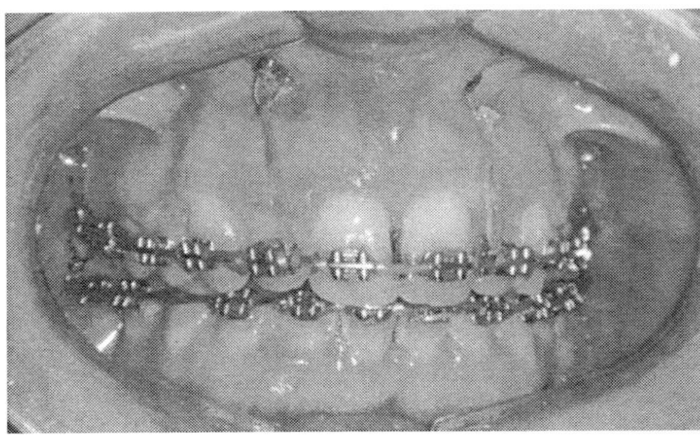

Figure 2. Intrution of anterior teeth with orthodontics mini-screws.

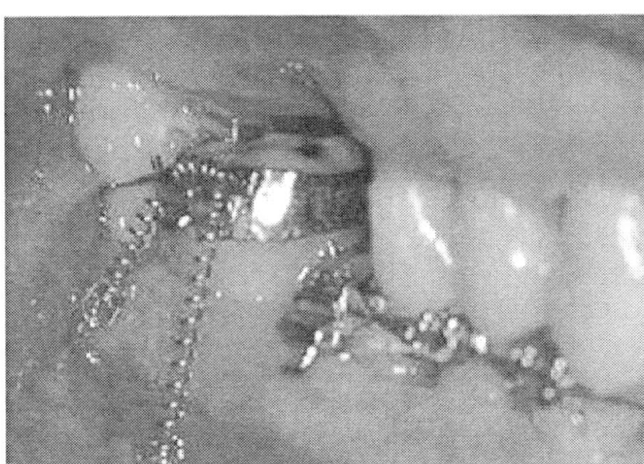

Figure 3. Intrusion of mandibalar molar with orthodontics mini-screws.

This chapter aims to highlight the influence of the oral and orthodontic load on surface properties of mini-screws. It focuses on the prevalence of use of mini-screws in accordance with clinical indications, location and duration of active treatment, and investigates the different histological reactions of peri-implant soft tissues and changes affecting the state of surface miniscrews collected after orthodontic treatment.

2. Mini-Screws As Orthodontic Anchorage

Ensuring proper anchorage is a major concern when orthodontic forces are applied. On the basis of Newton's third law, for every action there is an equal and opposite reaction, the impact of which is often undesirable during orthodontic treatment. "Thus, the orthodontist is constantly confronted with unwanted parasitic movements".

Only one anchorage system can effectively counter these unwanted movements. In some cases, anchorage control is difficult to maintain (Philippart et al., 2004). This is particularly true with adults, when there is a decrease in the number of teeth; when the alveolar ridges are more or less absorbed, when there is loss of *bone* density, or when a periodontal disease results in more or less important mobility. *In fact, clinical studies have shown that insufficient anchorage may jeopardize a successful result.*

Reliable and easy to implement anchoring systems are very important assests for orthodontists. Several systems implants of different designs have been suggested, leading to today miniscrews, which optimally meet the specifications required by orthodontists in anchorage (Philippart et al., 2004).

Most research on mini-screws involves clinical cases of little or no scientific value. A search on PubMed turned up a dozen randomized studies into mini-screws. Different teams (Melsen (2001), Frendenthaler (2001), Miyawaki (2003), Gelgor (2004), Wiechmann (2007), Cheng (2004), Park (2001), Kyung (61), Deguchi (2006), Sugawara (2004), Kuroda (2007), and Lin (2006) have helped develop valid clinical protocols and establish success rates that can be used as references.

On samples ranging from 15 to 227 miniscrews, the overall success rate varies between 75 and 93.4%. Weichmann et al. (2007) quickly discovered that mini-screws placed on the *mandible* lingual aspect all fail more or less early. He, therefore, eliminated this mini-screw site from his practice and was able to achieve a success rate of 97%.

The multidirectional forces generated by the tongue place lingually positioned mini-screws under constant stress and thus jeopardize their stability from the moment they are inserted. Lingual placement of mini-screws on the lower jaw has thus been eliminated from clinical protocols.

Furthermore, these studies have allowed matching miniscrew sizes and insertion sites. Surgical insertion has also been explored, but most emphasis has been placed on gradual mini-screw loading using traction auxiliaries. For a long time, research on the histological and chemical phenomena that result from *bone*-to-*implant contact* has occupied a greater place in orthodontics. Depending on the material used, operative techniques or protocols, there is a formation of a fibrous capsule of undifferentiated fibers; thickening of the capsule may lead to the expulsion of the implant. We speak of fibro-integration or osseo-integration which consists of the anatomic and direct functional junction between the remodeled living bone and the loaded implant surface, or mixed forms alternating areas of osseo-integration and fibrous encapsulation. Implants inserted in the edentulous areas are utilized to move teeth before rehabilitation. Orthodontic implants can be placed outside the arcades, retro molar areas, palate, the zygomatic arch, the nasal spine, symphysis and ramus. Healing process takes longer, and the cost of treatment is usually high. In their respective studies, Odman et al. (1994) and Kraut et al. (1988) carried out experiments involving tipping, torque and rotation, extrusion and intrusion with titanium implants placed in edentulous areas. Roberts et al. (1990) moved the molars toward edentulous areas, with implants installed in the retro-molar area. Higuchi et al. (1991) applied forces from 150 to 400g and achieved protraction, retraction and transverse changes, and the leveling of the whole arcade. The end of the 20th century marked a new area in implant technology; implants came in smaller size; were easy to place; and relatively cheap, Such factors made osteointegration redundant; reduced healing period, and allowed immediate loading. Over the years, researches have measured the breadth of applications enabled by these techniques. Among the most important advantages are mass retraction, molar uprighting and molar intrusion (Soulet, 2006).

3. Peri Implants Soft-Tissues

The soft tissues that surround dental implants are termed peri-implant mucosa. *The structure* and dimension of this *mucosa have* many features in *common* with those of the gingiva *around teeth.* Besides the biological width concept that controls the thickness of the soft tissue adjacent to both teeth and implants, there are also fundamental differences between the two tissue types.

Thus, the tooth roots are covered *with cementum* from which collagen fibers are oriented in a direction perpendicular to the longitudinal axis of the tooth and attach themselves to surrounding hard and soft tissues. The implant has no root and, hence, collagen fibers are not able to attach to the implant surface in the same way as the biological and mechanical attachment of teeth. In the peri-implant mucosa, the collagen fibers are aligned in different directions and in the tissues directly adjacent to the surface of the implant; the collagen fibers orient themselves parallel to the longitudinal axis of the implant (Figure 4, 5).

Nevertheless, the biological attachment formed by the barrier epithelium and the connective tissue part of the peri-implant mucosa provides an effective soft tissue seal to the oral environment. The integration of hard and soft tissues with implants is the result of a wound healing process. The tissue reactions that occur at recipient sites following implant placement include the formation of a blood clot that, within a few days, becomes infiltrated by vascular structures and numerous inflammatory cells to establish an early granulation tissue.

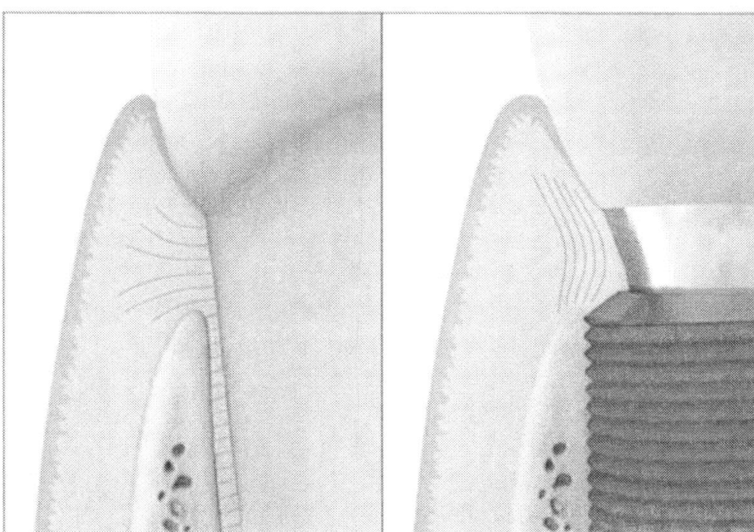

Figures 4 and 5. Orientation of collagen fibers at the joint: soft tissues/tooth soft tissues/ implant.

The continuation of the healing process involves the substitution of the granulation tissue by organized connective tissue from which bone formation occurs that eventually results in osseointegration.

The healing events in the mucosal compartment include the formation of a barrier epithelium adjacent to the implant and, apical to this epithelium, a connective tissue that integrates with the titanium surface and thereby prevents epithelial migration. The barrier epithelium and the connective tissue/implant interface establish the specific biological width of the peri-implant mucosa (Berglundh and Lindhe, 1996). The integration of hard and soft tissues with the implant device is a dynamic process that requires several weeks of healing.

4. Peri-Implantits Inflammation

Inflammatory lesions that develop in peri-implant tissues are collectively termed peri-implant disease. In accordance with the classification of periodontal disease around teeth, peri-implant disease includes two entities: peri-implant mucositis, which corresponds to gingivitis and peri-implantits, which corresponds to periodontitis. Thus, peri-implant mucositis is a condition that describes inflammation in the mucosa, while peri-implantits affects the supporting bone (Lindhe et al., 2008).

The detection of inflammation in the peri-implant mucosa requires probing to identify bleeding and/or suppuration. While the probing pocket depth (PPD) may vary around implants; such assessments are secondary to bleeding on probing (BoP). Sites with PPD $\geq$ 6 mm, however, may indicate pathology and should thus be examined meticulously. For the appraisal of peri-implantits, the detection of marginal bone loss in radiographs is also needed. In this context, it is important to distinguish between the bone remodeling that occurs early after implant installation and the loss of supporting bone that may be detected around implants during function. Thus, for appropriate evaluation of bone level changes around implants a reference radiograph, obtained directly after the delivery of the prosthesis, is required.

Peri-implantits lesions, in contrast to mucositis lesions, exhibit characteristics that are considerably different from their periodontal counterparts (Figure 6, 7). The inflammatory lesion in periodontitis around teeth is confined to the sub-epithelial connective tissue compartment of the gingiva and is separated from the alveolar bone by a 1mm-wide zone of dense connective tissue.

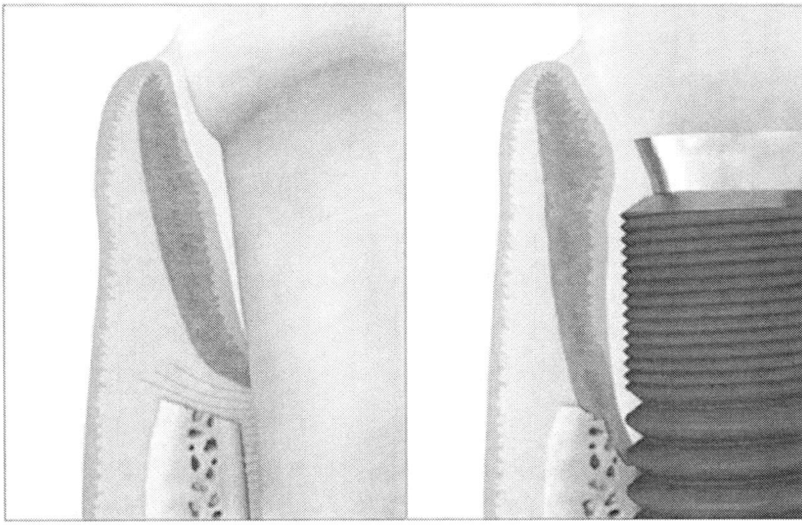

Figure 6 and 7. Parodontite lesion.

Furthermore, the pocket area is lined by a pocket epithelium, which in its most apical portion, is in contact with the root surface and thereby effectively walls off the biofilm of bacteria in the pocket.

The peri-implantits lesion also presents with a pocket compartment that contains bacteria. In contrast to the pocket epithelium in periodontitis, however, the corresponding epithelium of the peri-implantits lesion does not cover the entire extension of the pocket. As a consequence, the apical third of the inflamed tissue in the pocket is uncovered and in direct contact with the biofilm. Another difference in relation to periodontitis is the extension of the inflammatory lesion in peri-implantits. While the lesion in perio-dontitis is separated from the crestal bone by a zone of connective tissue, the lesion in peri-implantits extends to a position close to the bone surface. An understanding of these differences between periodontitis and peri-implantits is important in the selection of strategies for treatment of the disease.

Subjects with a high susceptibility to periodontitis are considered to be at a higher risk for peri-implantits (Heitz-Mayfield, 2008). Although all implant patients require sufficient follow-up and supportive therapy during maintenance, subjects susceptible to periodontitis should be provided with comprehensive infection control during follow-up in order to prevent peri-implant disease. Peri-implantits, as periodontitis around teeth, is more frequent among smokers than non-smokers.

As reported in clinical and experimental studies, implant surface characteristics are an additional risk factor for peri-implantits. Not only surface roughness but also surface composition appears to influence the onset and progression of peri-implantits. The design of the implant-supported prosthesis may be another risk factor for peri-implant disease. Access to infection control procedures performed by the patient and the dentist and/or dental hygienist must be provided in order to prevent inflammation in the peri-implant tissues.

5. The Corrosion Phenomenon

Corrosion, one of the phenomena that the biological environment is able to initiate, can cause a number of tissue reactions, which are histologically well codified. This is why the study of the compatibility of metals used with implants has been extensively developed.

To account for the mechanism of corrosion, several hypotheses have been put proposed. Crolet (1992), for example, speaks of "the myth of differential aeration" related to the accumulation in places clumps of plaque. He maintains that although this is not the main reason for corrosion, it would be a process of initiation. In aerated medium, the reduction of oxygen increases the pH favoring passivation, whereas in the anode regions, the hydrolysis of ions lowers the pH, and increases the acidity, which promotes corrosion.

This pH drop is added to that caused by micro-organisms of dental plaque. Indeed, micro-organisms secrete organic acids (lactic acid) that modify the local pH and may attack metals insufficiently resistant electrochemically or have suffered a mechanical fatigue developing in cracks and crevices in the metal surface, which will be a favorite location for microbial attack by anodic differential aeration (Picard, 1984).

This degradation, which can be chemical, electrochemical or biological, is a real economic problem. Its devastating effect leads all users of metals to predict a lifetime for metal parts and a cost for replacement and processing (Guyonnet et al., 2008). *There* are different *forms* of *corrosion*, which are more or less interrelated. *Uniform attack* is characterized by a chemical or electrochemical reaction while galvanic corrosion occurs when two dissimilar metals in contact with one another are placed in a corrosive environment or a conductive solution, which produces an electron flow between them; Crevice corrosion results from intense localized attack, usually associated with small volumes of stagnant solutions in shielded areas while the remaining surface experiences little or no damage. It is a form of galvanic corrosion due to impurities or inclusions in the alloy.

These phenomena may be exacerbated by oral polymetallism. Thermalionic, microbiological and enzymatic variations make the oral environment very favorable for the degradation of metallic materials (Grosgogeat et al., 2002). This is a form of localized corrosion due to fluctuations in concentration electrolytes or pH changes in a confined space, in addition to the effect of constraints imposed on the material (Greener 1971; Black, 1985).

Oral environment is favorable for the biodegradation of metals due to its chemical properties that accelerate the corrosion process. The *large population* of *bacteria* and *fungi* present in the oral environment may *accelerate* the *corrosion* of *orthodontic appliances*. In addition, orthodontic treatment may promote the formation of clusters of acido-genic biofilm, where the pH can be very acidic.

The tendency to dissolution of metals becomes very high in these areas. Bacterial colonization is at two levels: first, certain bacterial species can attack the metal and cause their dissolution and on the other hand, inorganic and organic acids from microbial metabolism may play a role in the degradation process. Thus, maintaining a good oral hygiene during orthodontic treatment minimizes the drop in pH and thus improves the corrosion behavior of alloys present in the mouth (Matasa, 1995; Richard, 1991). Inflammatory stress can also increase the corrosion of mini-screws, however, aggressive electrochemical conditions are necessary for the overall assessment of these effects (Messer et al., 2009). Corrosion can severely limit the fatigue life of the miniscrews.

The release of corrosion products *may* elicit an *adverse biological reaction* in the *host*; several authors have reported an increase in systemic and local concentrations of metals in connection with the metal of the mini-screws (Pazzaglia et al., 1986; Dorr et al., 1990).

There is no specific histological evidence that the slow release of metal species in relation to any metal implants accelerates corrosion and causes a reaction of peri-implant tissues that can be connected directly to identifiable products of corrosion (Urban et al., 1994).

The consequences of electrochemical corrosion in the oral cavity are related to the release, dissemination and storage of metal ions in the hard tissues (bones and teeth), soft tissue and fluids (saliva and blood).

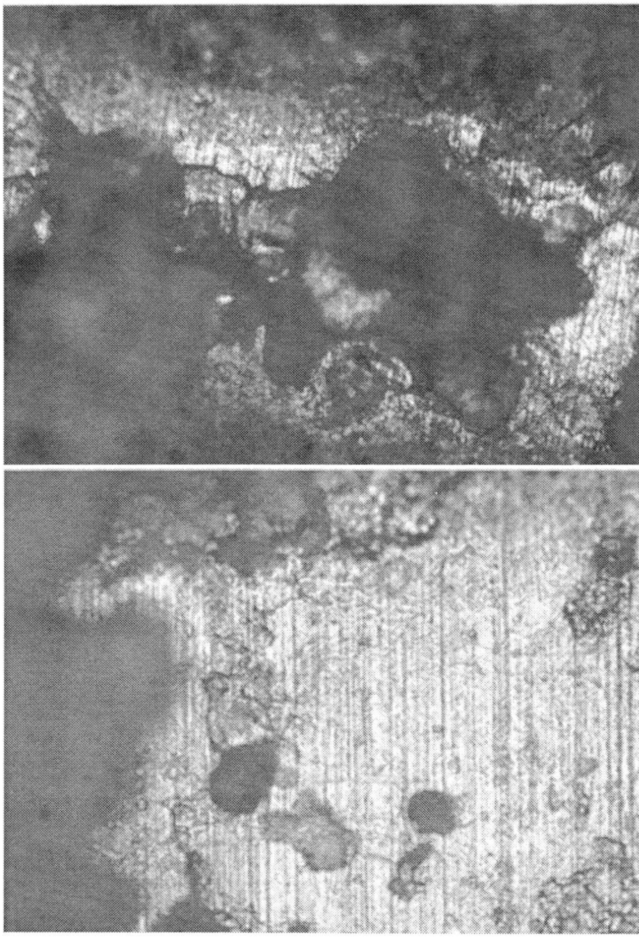

Figure 8 and 9. Optical microscopy views of miniscrew: extensive corrosion attacks with significant alloy destruction. Here the corrosion takes the form of crevices and deep pitting.

On the anodic metal, a total or partial destruction of the element may occur especially if it is buried (Renault et al., 2008). Corrosion products have been implicated in the onset of local pain and swelling in the region of mini-screws in the absence of infection.

The presence of corrosion and *wear products* found in *tissues surrounding* the mini-screws ultimately result in a *cascade* of *events* involving inflamemation and *leading* to bone loss (Park et al., 1992).

A few studies reported the release of metal ions from orthodontic appliances, the rate of which is *well below the daily dietary intake*. Nevertheless, some patients may be sensitive to nickel and have allergic reactions when exposed to alloys containing nickel (stainless steel and NiTi). Orthodontic treatment may even weaken the immune system and lower the tolerance for Ni (House et al., 2008).

The release of metal ions can also alter, irreversibly, the tooth enamel by the development of gray spots. Given the *current state* of *knowledge*, the effect of corrosion on the performance of orthodontic appliances, and on the health of patients, is poorly understood. More research with a particular focus on in vivo studies should be conducted to better understand the effects of corrosion (House et al., 2008).

6. Biocompatibility of Mini-Screws

Miniscrews like any other material placed in the human body must have good biological qualities. Compatibility is a term used to cover the mutual interaction between a surgical implant and its host. This term is used broadly to include the reactions of the tissue and its surroundings in its proximity and distance, as well as the effects of the human body on the implant itself.

The physico-chemical and biological properties of titanium *have* long *been* recognized. Titanium metal was first used in human medicine in orthopedic implants primarily for internal fixation and *prosthetic joints*. It was only in the early 70s that this harmless material was used in dental implant on account of its excellent corrosion resistance, biocompatibility and osseointegration behavior (Wirz, 1998).

Commercially pure titanium (CP Ti) is widely used as implant material because of its suitable mechanical properties and excellent biocompatibility. However, CP Ti has lower fatigue strength than titanium alloys. Titanium alloys can be used to overcome this disadvantage. However, the corrosion resistance of the mini-implant decreases when the alloy is used, favoring metal ion release, which has been associated with clinical implant failure, osteolysis, cutaneous allergic reactions, remote site accumulation, kidney lesion, cytotoxicity, hypersensitivity and carcinogenesis (Simon et al., 2005).

Electrochemical processes or mechanical surface treatment of implants all tend to get *a rough surface* to increase the microscopic bone-implant interface, so that the bone tissue can grow on an increased surface area of titanium oxide. The titanium surface that does not involve a special treatment is frequently associated with a smooth surface. A perfectly smooth implant surface does not lead to osseointegration (Wennerberg et al., 2000). The shaping of titanium mini-screws creates an irregular surface parallel to the turns of implant body. These geometric defects are of 2 types: a difference in shape due to deformation during *machine operation*, tool operation, or the guide to the shaping of the mini-screws or undulations due to the vibration of the tool or part of it (Renault, 2008).

Mini-screws most often contain titanium. More precisely, they are made of a titanium, aluminum and vanadium alloy (TiAl6V4), which is stronger than commercially pure titanium. There also exist several systems using surgical steel.

Titanium is, however, extremely very sensitive to corrosion which result in both particles of titanium oxide and titanium alloys. Wear/corrosion occurs as result of friction at the level of articulatory surfaces, the micro-motion of intra-osseous portion, of the abrasion surrounding tissue and of metal-to-metal contact. The biocompatibility of each metal is governed by the degree of corrosion and toxicity of metal ions released. Titanium exhibits a *good biocompatibility* because of its excellent corrosion resistance and very low ions release, related to the apparent absence of biological metal effects. This finding was confirmed in a number of clinical and experimental studies, all of which favor a minimal tissue response to this metal (Muster et al., 1999; Liliane et al., 2007).

In general, the surface of the mini-screws in direct contact with host tissues plays a critical role in determining biocompatibility. Particular attention must be given to the stability of the surface of these biomaterials because its composition and structure are commonly affected by the tissue response after implantation. For example, the inflammatory response and contact with the oral environment may alter the surface characteristics of biomaterials (Nanci et al., 1998).

7. A Study Conducted at Casablanca School of Dentistry

The present study aimed to investigate the different histological reactions of peri-implant soft tissues and the changes affecting the surface condition of recovered mini-screws patients following orthodontic treatment (Sebbar et al., 2010; Sebbar et al., 2011).

7.1. Subjects, Materials and Method

The sample consisted of 13 patients following treatment at Casablanca orthodontics center in Casablanca; 28 *mini-screws* (Dual-Top Anchor System; Lotus Orthodontics, Korea) *were* inserted for various orthodontic indications (ingression, anterior retraction, decrease in mass, asymmetry correction, etc.). The mini-screws were of different diameters and lengths. Different practitioners placed all mini-screws under the same conditions. These mini-screws were loaded immediately after installation, using a screwdriver supplied by the manufacturer.

An observation sheet was completed for each patient including patient identification, orthodontic diagnosis, treatment schedule and mini-screws insertion; the observation sheet serves to explain to the patients what the treatment will consist of by showing them examples of mini-screws and by describing how they function (indication, location, date of insertion of the mini-screws and the date removal thereof). Data collection was performed on an individual record for each variable: a file for histology and another one for the study of the state of the surface.

Table 1 describes our sample based on a history of periodontal disease, indications, location and duration of active treatment. Patients were informed about the procedure prior to surgery, and the problems that mini-screws can give rise to during malocclusion treatment; at the same time, they were informed about alternative treatment options.

The locations of mini-screws were chosen after a detailed analysis of treatment goals, a careful historical and radiographical evaluation. The size and the diameter of the mini-screws were chosen according to anatomical site, depending on the quantity and quality of the bone.

A histological examination of our sample was performed in a private histology laboratory. Each mini-screw was removed using a self-drilling procedure under local anesthesia.

Samples were placed in individual boxes containing a mounting product (the formalin) and sent later to the laboratory for a histological examination. The examination allowed exploring the different histological reactions of peri-implant tissues. Patients were informed about the purpose of the study, the procedure prior to surgery; written consent was obtained.

Table 1. List of mini-screws used for orthodontic anchorage, including information on the indication for use, location and duration of active treatment

Miniscrews N°	Indication	Localization	Duration	History of periodontal disease
1	Intrusion	Palate between 16 and 17	12 months	No
2	Anterior Retraction	Vestibular between 15 and16	12 months	No
3	Anterior Retraction	Vestibular between 15 and 16	7 months	No
4	Anterior Retraction	Vestibular between 45 and 46	14 months	No
5	Intrusion	Vestibular between 32 and 33	4 months	No
6	Intrusion	Palatal / distal 16	8 months	No
7	Anterior Retraction	Vestibular between 26 and 27	12 months	No
8	Intrusion	Vestibular between 26 and 27	6 months	No
9	Intrusion	Palatal between 16 and 17	24 months	No
10	Anterior Retraction	Vestibular between 25 and 26	7months	No

Miniscrews N°	Indication	Localization	Duration	History of periodontal disease
11	Intrusion	Vestibular / Mesial 26	28months	Yes
12	Anterior Retraction	Vestibular / Mesial 15	11 months	Yes
13	Intrusion	Vestibular / Mesial	28months	Yes
14	Intrusion	Vestibular between 14 and 15	10months	No
15	Anterior Retraction	Vestibular between 25 and 26	12months	No
16	Anterior Retraction	Vestibular between 15 and 16	19months	No
17	Lifting of Overbite	Vestibular between 11 and 12	9months	Yes
18	Anterior Retraction	Vestibular between 15 and 16	6months	No
19	Correction of asymmetry	Vestibular / Mesial of 45	12months	No
20	Intrusion	Palatal /distal of 26	28months	Yes
21	Intrusion	Palatal between 15 and 16	10months	No

Table 1. (Continued)

Miniscrews N°	Indication	Localization	Duration	History of periodontal disease
22	Intrusion	Vestibular /Mesial of 16	8months	No
23	Anterior Retraction	Vestibular between 16 and 17	12months	No
24	Intrusion	Palatal between 15 and 16	14months	No
25	Lifting of overbite	Vestibular between 21 and 22	9months	Yes
26	Intrusion	Vestibular between 26 and 27	24 months	No
27	Anterior Retraction	Vestibular between 15 and 17	17 months	Yes
28	Intrusion	Vestibular/Mesial of 16	28 months	Yes

All the miniscrews used were recovered and placed in self-sealed plastic boxes, containing all the information already listed on the computer sheet. A new miniscrew provided by the manufacturer served as control. Due to variations in use, differences in the quality life of minscrews, and the insertion of these miniscrews in different patients, we included samples from the same manufacturer to control these different variables. After cleaning the miniscrews with acetone, they were examined under an optical microscope (Leica DM2500 M) and observed from three perspectives (x5, x10, x20) in order to study the machining defects and changes affecting the state of surface and compare the results of observations with those of the control miniscrew. The study was conducted at Casablanca Dental Laboratory of Sciences.

7.2. Results

The 28 miniscrews were placed at different sites. 14 mini-screws were used for molar intrusion, 11 mini-screws for retraction of anterior teeth, 2 mini-screws were shown to raise an incisor overbite and one mini-screw was used to correct asymmetry.

21 mini-screws were placed in the buccal region while 7 mini-screws had a palatal location. 3 mini-screws were placed in front and 25 mini-screws had a posterior position. 25 mini-screws were used in the maxilla and 3 mini-screws were placed in the mandible. 3 mini-screws were used for a period of 1 to 6 months, 9 mini-screws for a period of 6 to 12 months and 16 mini-screws for 12 months or more.

Sample harvesting was performed without any particular complication and with no undesirable impact on the different sites. Postoperative follow-up of the sample sites evidenced complete healing of the peri-implant tissue with no sign of inflammation or bleeding.

All samples exhibited signs of inflammation. Every tissue fragment displayed moderately or highly inflamed surface epithelium and underlying connective tissue. The surface epithelium lining was frequently papillomatous and edematous. The connective tissue contained collagen fibers with an inflammatory infiltrate comprising vascular structures and inflammatory cells in varying quantities depending upon the degree of inflammation.

These inflammatory cells were primarily lymphocytes, histocytes and plasma cells that dominated the lesion, alongside the occasional granulocyte (Figure 10 and 11).

With respect to the findings of the histologic analysis of the samples taken in the vicinity of miniscrews # 11 and 20, we observed only a superficial epithelial covering and no chorion; the sampling was not performed deep enough to include the connective tissue underlying the epithelium. The presence of inflammation in all patients with and without a history of periodontal disease suggests there is no correlation between inflammation of the peri-implant soft tissue and peri-odontal disorders.

A similar observation can be made regarding the use of miniscrews since signs of inflammation were present in all patients irrespective of the duration of usage (long or short) of the implants. The findings of the present study demonstrate that the peri-implant mucosa around the vestibular sites subjected to daily brushing for dental plaque was clinically inflamed as compared to palatal sites.

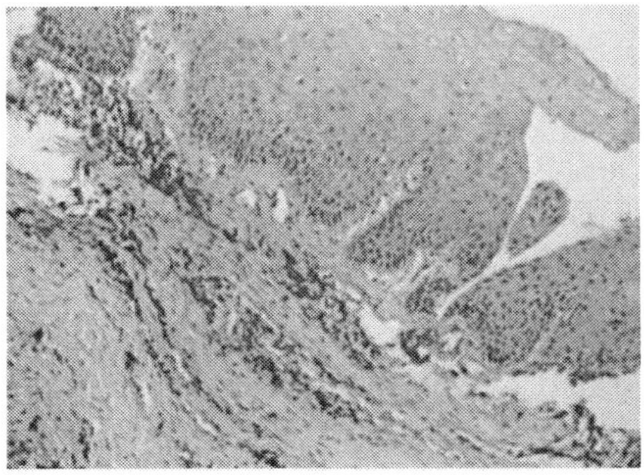

Figure 10. Malpighian mucosa with papillomatous surface. The chorion is edematous, congestive and highly inflamed and has been heavily infiltrated by lymphoplasmocytes.

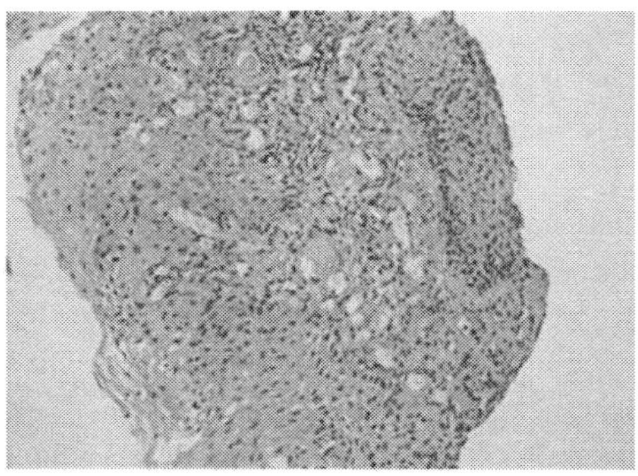

Figure 11. Malpighian mucosa with papillomatous surface, edematous and highly inflamed chorion containing lymphoplasmocytes.

We can thus conclude that the position of the miniscrew (vestibular or palatal) had no influence on the presence or absence of inflammation. The miniscrews used in this study were made of titanium or, more accurately, of a titanium-alloy containing aluminum and vanadium (TiA16V4). All miniscrews were fitted and removed without breakage or bending. We noted that the miniscrews were easily removed, thus suggesting absence of osteointegration. After removal, the miniscrews were examined by means of an optical microscope (113) in order to determine their surface status. Observations were made across the entire surface of the miniscrew using three magnifying lenses (5, 10, 20). Image magnification (10, 20) allowed us to better visualize the surface status and pinpoint the various alterations affecting the miniscrew surface.

Despite a smooth appearance to the naked eye, the control miniscrew had surface milling and polishing defects in the form of scratches, which can serve as a starting point for electrochemical attacks. Observations under optical microscopy evidenced signs of corrosion in the form of pitting and crevices, principally at the site of the manufacturing defects (Figure 12 and 13). Optic microscopy images of the retrieved miniscrews indicated considerable variability in the surface state. Miniscrews placed in the mouth emphasize their manufacturing defects due to the widening of the scratches due to corrosive attack in the form of pitting and crevices. This inevitably results in a damaged passivation layer following destruction of the protective titanium dioxide film on the surface of the alloy (Figures 14 and 15).

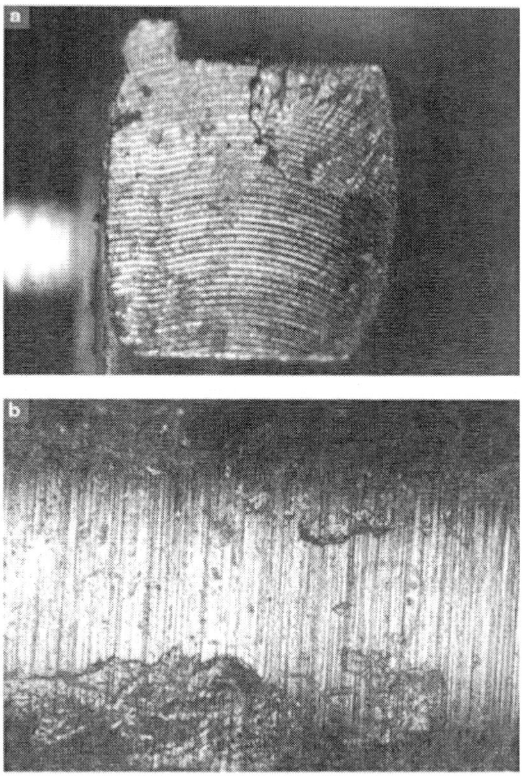

Figure 12. Optical microscopy views of the control miniscrew showing a highly irregular surface with manufacturing defects and alloy impurities: a: control miniscrew, magnification 5; b: control miniscrew, magnification 10.

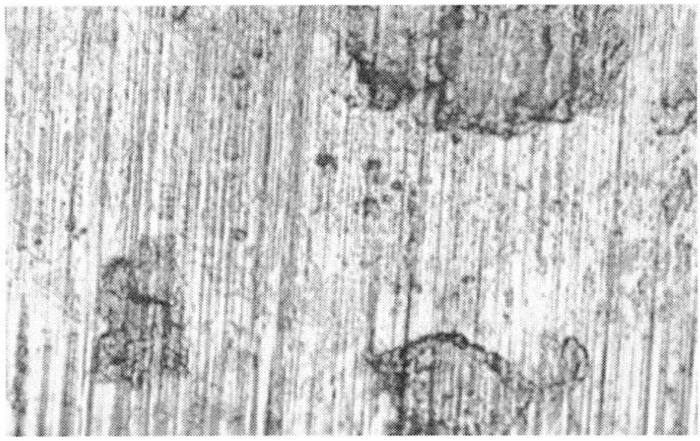

Figure 13. Control miniscrew, magnification 20. Optical microscopy views of control miniscrew: irregular surface showing manufacturing defects and alloy impurities. Defects vary in size but can be seen over the entire miniscrew surface.

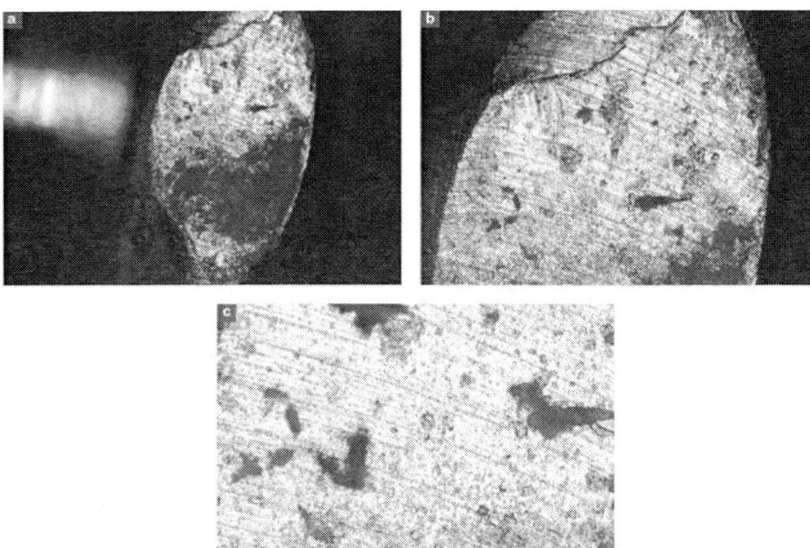

Figure 14. Optical microscopy views showing the head of miniscrew No. 18: Visible pitting and crevice corrosion. Attacks were more prevalent than on the control miniscrew. We noted more signs of crevice corrosion than pitting: a: miniscrew No. 18, magnification 5; b: miniscrew No. 18, magnification 10; c: miniscrew No. 18, magnification 20.

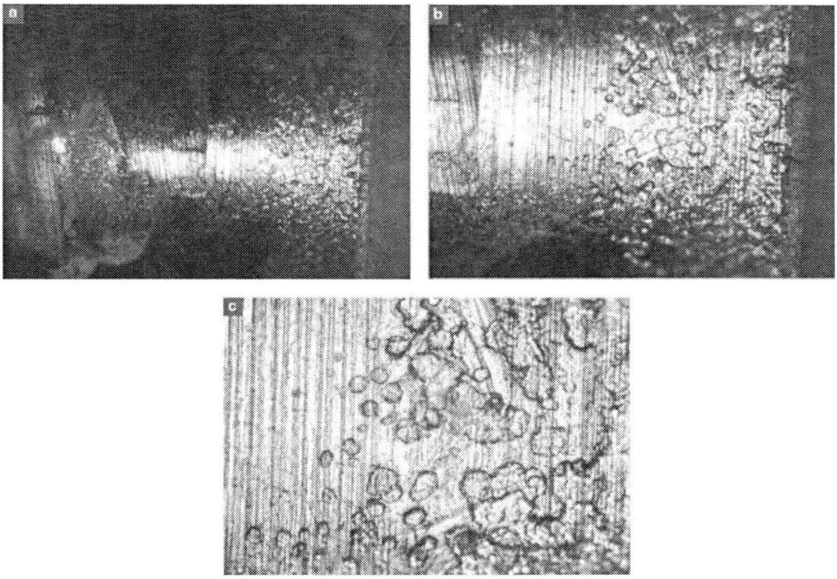

Figure 15. Optical microscopy views of miniscrew No. 20: pitting corrosion due to manufacture defects: a: miniscrew No. 20, magnification 5; b: miniscrew No. 20, magnification 10; c: miniscrew No. 20, magnification 20.

All the specimens exhibited loss of gloss and polish and, consequently, a dull surface. Localized pitting was the most frequent form of corrosion observed in our sample.

7.3. Discussion

7.3.1. Histologic Analysis

Histologic analysis of peri-implant soft tissue revealed that the mucosa samples taken around the miniscrews comprised sur- face epithelium and underlying connective tissue displaying signs of inflammation of varying intensity.

Berglundh et al. (1991) compared the structure and composition of peri-implant mucosa and clinically sound gingival margin (in the beagle dog). Histologic analysis evidenced, for all the tissue samples, the presence of keratinized oral epithelium and a roughly 2 mm junction epithelium. The height of the supracrestal gingival connective tissue was approximately 1 mm. The collagen fiber bundles were fan-shaped, originating at the cellular root cementum. Titanium implants showed no traces of cementum and the collagen fiber bundles of the peri-implant mucosa originated at the surface of the bone (Berglundh et al., 1985).

Other histologic assessments performed in dogs have shown that fixation of the implant is provided by a biocompatible, healthy and functional epithelial junction similar to that of teeth. Further in the apical direction, an area of junction tissue is located between the epithelial junction and the bone. The junction tissue fibers are aligned parallel to the implant contrary to the situation with teeth where the junction fibers are inserted at the cementum layer and are perpendicular to the root (Polat-Ozsoy et al., 2009).

Ultra structural analysis by transmission electron microscopy revealed that fibroblasts at the interface had a flat and elongated appearance in both vertical and horizontal directions (Moon et al., 1999, Abrahamsson et al., 2002).

Qualitative analysis of the underlying connective tissue at the junction epithelium in the supracrestal location showed that the peri-implant mucosa contains more collagen and fewer fibroblasts than corresponding gingival connective tissue.

Berglundh et al. (2004) made a histologic analysis, in man, of biopsies taken around implants exhibiting signs of inflammation and bone loss. Their observations show that:

- keratinized epithelium continued into the epithelium;
- the apical section of the pocket epithelium was thin and ulcerated;
- the connective tissue had been infiltrated by inflammatory cells extending further apically than the pocket epithelium;
- the infiltrated connective tissue contained collagen fibers, vascular structures and inflammatory cells;
- at the margins of the lesion, the tissue had been infiltrated by lymphocytes and plasma cells (60%). Vessels were few but broad, occupying the central area of the marginal portion of the lesion;
- the inflammatory cells and the vessels were preponderant in the lesion; plasma cells and polymorphonuclears (PMN) were found not only in the pocket epithelium and underlying connective tissue but also in the perivascular compartments at a distance from the implant-bearing surface.

In our study, we found the same components in the peri- implant mucosa with a moderately or very inflamed surface epithelium and connective tissue. The epithelial surface coating was often papillomatous and edematous and the connective tissue contained collagen fibers with an inflammatory infiltrate consisting of vascular structures and inflammatory cells in different quantities according to the degree of inflammation.

The anatomical localization and duration of usage of the mini-screw were factors, which affected the survival rate of the implants. Miniscrews placed in the alveolar mucosa triggered considerable tissue irritation and inflammation, which could account for miniscrew failure, whereas implants inserted in the attached gingiva displayed a success rate of over 90% (Kuroda et al., 2002).

The mandibular failure rate was found to be similar to that of the maxilla, even though the mandibular cortex is thinner than the maxillary. The mandibular failure rate could be related to the narrowness of the attached gingiva in the posterior region, which complicates implant insertion at this site (Deguchi et al., 2006).

In order to ensure maximum stability, the miniscrew should be positioned in regions of greater soft and hard tissue thickness. Nevertheless, thin peri-implant soft tissue is less subject to inflammation (Deguchi et al., 2006).

In patients with no attached gingiva, implants need to be placed more coronally with greater gingival support. With respect to palatal sites, the thickness of the soft tissue is more vital than that of the cortical bone. It is advisable to place implants close to the cemento-enamel junction on the palatal aspect where the soft tissue is thicker (Kim et al., 2006).

Ericsson et al. (1995) have shown that the peri-implant mucosa at sites subjected to thorough daily monitoring of dental plaque during biopsy was clinically inflammation-free and that the connective tissue lateral to the junction epithelium was devoid of aggregations of inflammatory cells.

Moreover, the termination of the dental plaque-monitoring program led to the aggregation of large quantities of dental plaque and tartar around the head of the miniscrews. In this context, the biopsies harvested from the implant sites after 9 months of plaque formation revealed the presence of an infiltrate within the marginal portion of the peri-implant region.

This infiltrate was found both in sites which had been sub- jected to dental plaque monitoring and at sites where dental plaque had been allowed to form over a period of 9 months. These findings matched those of our own study since inflamed infiltrate was observed at all the miniscrew implant sites, both at sites subjected to plaque monitoring and at those, which were not.

It is suggested that this infiltration is the result of the efforts of the host to eliminate the bacteria present in the peri-implant soft tissue (Ericsson et al., 1995). The peri-implant soft tissue responds to the formation of 3 weeks of dental plaque by developing an inflamed lesion. Given that these two types of lesion were of the same size and composition, one can conclude that the peri-implant gingiva and mucosa share the same ability to counter the formation of dental plaque (Buser et al., 1992).

Prolonged accumulation of dental plaque triggers the devel- opment of an inflammatory cell inflammation in the peri- implant gingiva and mucosa. The two infiltrates share the same characteristics although they are more prevalent in the peri-implant mucosa than in the gingival tissue. These findings suggest that the gingival defense mechanisms can be as efficacious as those of the peri-implant mucosa in preventing the apical migration of bacteria from the pocket (Berglundh et al., 2004)

If the patient presents an infection or general symptoms such as fever, prolonged discomfort due to the orthodontic force and involvement of the adjacent periodontal attachments, the orthodontic miniscrew should be promptly removed.

7.3.2. Miniscrew Surface

Miniscrew surfaces are subject to corrosion following contact with the electrolyte composition of biological fluids. Surfaces are much more rapidly corroded when miniscrews are loaded while in service. Observation under optical microscopy evidenced signs of corrosion in the form of pitting or crevices principally on account of milling defects. Corrosion not only alters the nature of the surface but also the resistance and other properties of the material. In addition, products of corrosion can be released into neighboring tissues, inducing local and systemic reactions (Morais et al., 2007).

The ideal biomaterial for miniscrew implants should exhibit excellent corrosion resistance, biocompatibility and sufficient mechanical strength to enable orthodontic miniscrews to withstand the torsional forces to which they are subjected during insertion and removal. Though miniscrews often break at the neck in a clinical setting, such fractures are often the result of miniscrew design. The study by Lijima et al. (2008) focused on the connection between the microstructure of the alloys used in miniscrews and torsional stress rather than on the morphological factors involved in design.

Lijima et al. (2008) used four miniscrews of different brands and diameters. The composition of each miniscrew was determined by X-ray fluorescence. Mean moment and torsion angle values were then measured for each tested miniscrew. Results showed that two miniscrews were made of pure titanium whilst the two others also contained small amounts of vanadium, aluminum, iron and manganese.

Addition of these particles to the titanium (titanium alloy) significantly improved both the performance and the mechanical properties of the miniscrews, as well as their biocompatibility.

To determine the optimum safety factor for miniscrew implants, variations in mechanical properties and forms of deterioration such as torsional fatigue during tooth displacements or corrosion of fitted implants, must be considered (Lijima et al., 2008). Studies on retrieved miniscrew implants have been attracting growing interest in recent years in the area of dental materials on account of the focus on analyses of performance according to the environment in which the material is used. The drafting of international standards regarding retrieved orthopedic device analysis clearly indicates how important this method is when studying how materials behave.

Eliades et al. (2000) recovered NiTi arch wires from patients undergoing orthodontic treatment. These arch wires were then observed using optical and electron microscopy so as to determine their composition and the micro morphological surface changes occurring in the oral environment.

Optical microscopy revealed that the studied surfaces were partially covered with small patches of amorphous precipitants and areas of accumulated microcrystalline particles. Electron microscopy highlighted significant morphological variations compared to control samples, with the formation, after 2 months exposure in the mouth, of a surface biofilm and the presence of transitional zones between the unaffected areas of metal and the surface of the biofilm. The unaffected metal surface was smooth and displayed less pitting. The organic constituents of this biofilm were amide, alcohol and carbonate, whereas the main elements observed were crystals of Na, K, Cl, Ca and Ca-P (Eliades et al., 2000). In a similar study, Eliades et al. (2009) analyzed 11-retrieved miniscrew implants used in various orthodontic indications. The samples were used for an average active treatment time ranging between 3.5 and 17.5 months and removed with no sign of failures such as peri-implant soft-tissue inflammation, implant mobility or premature loss. Miniscrews matched by brand, type and size served as controls. All miniscrews were examined under stereomicroscopy to detect possible microscopic cracks. The structure of both retrieved and control miniscrews was analyzed by high-resolution X-ray computer tomography (CT). 2D and 3D reconstructions were then obtained to study the surface-loading pattern of miniscrews using cone-beam reconstruction and 3D creation software (Skyscan) [3]. The miniscrews were studied under electron microscopy to determine their morphological status. In addition, the retrieved and control miniscrews were assessed by energy dispersive X-ray microanalysis to determine their chemical composition (Eliades et al., 2009).

Results showed significant changes in miniscrew surfaces including adsorption and formation of a calcified layer due to contact of the implant with blood and tissue fluids. Optical microscopy showed loss of gloss with variable discoloring. Scanning electron microscopy and X-ray microanalysis revealed morphological changes with layers of sodium, potassium, chlorine, iron, calcium and phosphorus deposited on the miniscrew surface (Eliades et al., 2009). Two-dimensional micro tomography X-ray images reconstructing the longitudinal cross-section of a control miniscrew showed no defects in the form of pores or cracks due to surface loading in the mouth. Chemical analysis by electron surface microanalysis (EDS) indicated that miniscrew implant composition was similar to that of standard titanium alloy.

(Ti6Al4V). This analysis also suggested that calcium and iron precipitates had been induced by contact of the miniscrew with blood and biological fluids (Eliades et al., 2000). Surface characterization of retrieved miniscrews revealed an ageing process, as seen in numerous biomaterials ranging from polymers (Eliades et al., 1999) to orthodontic alloys, which basically involves the adsorption of protein layers which later become calcified and precipitate as phosphorus and calcium. The difference between retrieved oral-placed and tissue-placed material could reside in the iron composition when biomaterial surface comes into contact with blood.

Oral placement of miniscrews causes several phenomena:

- pH reduction during the initial exudative phases;
- cell activation, including for granulocytes, neutrophils and macrophages;
- release of proteins, enzymes and oxidative agents, which could significantly modify the implant's surface reactivity (Eliades et al., 1999).

Prolonged exposure of miniscrews in the mouth generates harder and more calcified precipitates than does shorter exposure length. Depending on patient and oral conditions, the metal surface is covered with a layer of protein, which conceals the surface topography of the alloy, the extent of the protein varying according to the conditions prevailing in the mouth of each patient (Hanning et al., 1999).

This surface layer significantly alters the morphology, surface composition and electronic reactivity of the implant. Mineralized areas can serve as a protection shielding the alloy substrate, particularly if pH or corrosion levels are low [(Oshida et al., 1992).

The key advantage of Ti alloys is the rapid formation of a dense and amorphous film of passive titanium dioxide (Eliades, 1999). Stress exerted on a miniscrew during healing can have severe adverse effects, depending on the duration of the stress.

We are of the opinion that poorly inserted miniscrews respond by developing reparative fibrous tissue.

Implant micro movement is an important factor in bone regeneration and has a much greater influence on bone healing and the properties of biomaterials (Eliades et al., 2000). In the absence of micro-movements, osseo-integration of the bone-biomaterial interface is more likely to be linked to potential inherent bone healing than to a single phenomenon induced by the biomaterial of which the implant is made. Han et al. (2002) studied surface states of miniscrews (both the submerged and visible degments) retrieved after oral placement ranging from 18 months to 4 years and 4 months.

Scanning electron microscopy performed on retrieved miniscrew surfaces showed major build-ups. Surface electron analysis (EDS) demonstrated that this build-up was made up of carbon and oxide. The organic substances consisted of dental plaque and corrosion products. Following ultrasonic cleansing, the EDS spectra showed that the miniscrew surfaces were made of titanium. The already-existing scratches now seemed to be deeper and new flaws were visible on the miniscrew surface. The surface of the as-received miniscrews revealed parallel milling scars around the circumference of the screws (Han et al., 2002).

More surface changes were observed on the embedded part of the miniscrew compared with the non-embedded section, thus accounting for the high incidence of breakage of the former. Patterson and Johns (1992) looked into fatigue-resistance of miniscrews and concluded that applying appropriate torque made for a longer miniscrew lifespan. Changes in miniscrew surfaces can result in instability. Surface modifications to retrieved miniscrews are difficult to explain (Schliephake et al., 1993).

In their study, Rangert and Langer (1995) found that miniscrew failures were caused by fatigue. Another study by Glauser et al. (2005) showed the presence of linear scoring pointing to the development of fatigue cracks, probably induced by repeated traction stresses. These cracks went on to spread over the entire implant surface (Basten et al., 1996)

Conclusion

Due to large variation in our sample (the site of implantation, type of mini-screws and surgical orthodontic movement desired, the amount of force applied and the use of immediate loading), findings of the study are quite limited. The present study demonstrated that ethical issues and human biopsies are generally more subject to differences with regards to the parameters influencing other tissue reactions. Therefore, interpretations in terms of the tissue responses should approached with caution.

Despite a smooth appearance to the *naked eye,* the mini-screws all *had* crack-like surface manufacturing. Electrochemical tests have showed that after use, *corrosion* can be concentrated locally to *form* a *pit* or *crack.* Consequently, an improvement of the surface *can improve* its corrosion resistance. The use of mini-screws in selected appropriate cases is a predictable and precise technique for peri-implant soft tissues in humans.

The patients' number and mini-screws analyzed in this study *were too small* to be representative*;* more studies involving *larger number of patients and mini-screws* are necessary.

References for Abstract

[1] Riendeau. F. Ancrage orthodontique intra-osseux à l'aide d'implants palatins. *J. Dent. Québec.* 2003; 40:293-296.

[2] Massif. L, L. Frapier. Utilisation clinique des minivis en orthodontie. *Encycl Méd Chir Odontologie/Orthopédie Dentofaciale*, 2006; 23-492-A-17.

[3] Davarpanah. M, Caraman. M. L'apport de l'ancrage squelettique en orthodontie. *Act. Odont. Stomatol.* 2007; 237:41-58.

[4] Philippart F, Philippart-Rochaix M. "Les minivis" : un concept d'ancrage orthodontique. *International Orthodontics* 2004; 2:319-330.

[5] Cornelis. M, Scheffler. N. Systematic review of the experimental use of temporary skeletal anchorage devices in orthodontics. *Am. J. Orthod. Dentofacial Orthop*. 2007; 131(4 Suppl): S52-8.

[6] Melsen B, CostaA. Immediate loading of implants used for orthodontic anchorage. *Clin. Orthod. Res.* 2000; 3:23-8.

[7] Buchter A, Wiechmann D. Load-related bone modelling at the interface of orthodontic micro-implants. *Clin. Oral Impl. Res.* 2006; 17: 714-722.

[8] Kim. J, Ahn. S. Histomorphometric and mechanical analyses of the drill-free screw as orthodontic anchorage. *Am. J. Orthod. Dentofacial Orthop.* 2005; 128:190-4.
[9] Oyonarte. R, Pilliar. R. Peri-implant bone response to orthodontic loading: Part 1. A histomorphometric study of the effects of implant surface design. *Am. J. Orthod. Dentofacial Orthop.* 2005; 128:173-81).
[10] Oyonarte. R, Pilliar. R. Peri-implant bone response to orthodontic loading: Part 2. Implant surface geometry and its effect on regional bone remodelling. *Am. J. Orthod. Dentofacial Orthop.* 2005;128:182-9.
[11] Naim S, Gregoire G. Importance de l'état de surface dans l'approche de la biocompatibilité d'un biomatériau. *J. Biomat. Dent.* 1998; 13:89-104.

References

Abrahamsson I, Zitzmann NU, Berglundh T, Linder E, Wennerberg A, Lindhe J. The mucosal attachment to titanium implants with different surface characteristics: an experi- mental study in dogs. *J. Clin. Periodontol* 2002; 29 (5):448–55.

Basten CH, Nicholls JI, Daly CH, Taggart R. Load fatigue performance of two implant- abutment combinations. *Int. J. Oral Maxillofac Implants* 1996; 11(4):522–8.

Black J. 'Metallic Ion Release and its relationship to Oncogenesis' In Fitzgerald RH Jr (ed): The Hip, St. Louis, Mosby, 1985:199-213.

Berglundh, T. Lindhe, J. Dimensions of the periimplant mucosa. Biological width revisited. *J. Clin. Periodontol.* 1996; 23: 971-973.

Berglundh T, Gislason O, Lekholm U. Histopathological observations of human periim- plantitis lesions. *J. Clin. Periodontol.* 2004;31(5):341–7.

Berglundh T, Lindhe J, Ericsson I, Marinello CP, Liljenberg B, Thomsen P. The soft tissue barrier at implants and teeth. *Clin. Oral Implants Res.* 1991; 2 (2):81-90.

Berglundh T, Lindhe J, Marinello CP, Ericsson I. soft tissue reaction to de novo plaque formation at implants and teeth: an experimental study in the dog. *Clin. Oral Implants Res.* 1992; 3:1-8.

Buchter A, Wiechmann D. Load-related bone modelling at the interface of orthodontic micro-implants. *Clin. Oral Impl. Res.* 2006;17: 714-722.

Buser D, Weber HP, Donath K, Fiorellini JP, Paquette DW, Williams RC. Soft tissue reactions to non-submerged unloaded titanium implants in beagle dogs. *J. Periodontol.* 1992;63 (3):225–35.

Cheng SJ, Tseng IY, Lee JJ, Kok SH. A prospective study of the risk factors associated with failure of mini-implants used for orthodontic anchorage. Int. *J. Oral Maxillofac Implants* 2004;19(1):100-106.

Cornelis. M, Scheffler. N. Systematic review of the experimental use of temporary skeletal anchorage devices in orthodontics. *Am. J. Orthod. Dentofacial Orthop.* 2007; 131(4 Suppl): S52-8.

Crolet J.-L. Biocorrosion : régulation du pH par les bactéries sulfato-réductrices. *Matériaux et Techniques* 1992; 9 –10: 71 – 77.

Davarpanah. M, Caraman. M. L'apport de l'ancrage squelettique en orthodontie. *Act. Odont. Stomatol.* 2007; 237: 41-58.

Deguchi T, Nasu M, Murakami K, Yabuuchi T. Quantitative evaluation of cortical bone thickness with computed tomographic scanning for orthodontic implants. *Am. J. Orthod. Dentofacial Orthop.* 2006; 129(6):721.e7-721.e12.

Dorr LD, Bloebaum R, Emmanual J, Meldrum R. Histologic, biochemical, and ion analysis of tissue and fluids retrieved during total hip arthroplasty. *Clin. Orthop.* 1990; 261: 82- 95.

Eliades T. Passive film growth on titanium alloys: physicochemical and biologic considera- tions. *Int. J. Oral. Maxillofac Implants* 1997;12: 621–7.

Eliades T, Eliades G, Athanasiou AE, Bradley TG. Surface characterization of retrieved NiTi orthodontic archwires. *Eur. J. Orthod.* 2000;22:317–26.

Eliades G, Eliades T, Vavuranakis M. General aspects of biomaterials' surface alterations following exposure to biological fluids. In: Eliades G., Eliades T., Brantley WA., Watts DC. (Eds.), Dental materials in vivo: aging and related phenomena. *Quintessence*, Chicago, 2000: 33-23.

Eliades T, Zinelis S, Papadopoulos M, Eliades G. Characterization of retrieved orthodontic miniscrew implants. *Am. J. Orthod. Dentofacial Orthop.* 2009;135: 10.e1–7.

Eliades T, Eliades G, Watts DC. Structural conformation of in vitro and in vivo-aged orthodontic elastomeric modules. *Eur. J. Orthod.* 1999; 6: 649–58.

Ericsson I, Persson LG, Berglundh T, Marinello CP. Different types of inflammatory reactions in peri-implant soft tissues. *J. Clin. Periodontol.* 1995; 22: 255-261.

Freudenthaler JW, Haas R, Bantleon HP. Bicortical titanium screws for critical orthodontic anchorage in the mandible: a preliminary report on clinical applications. *Clin. Oral Implants. Res*. 2001; 12 (4):358-363.

Gelgör IE, Büyükyilmaz T, Karaman AI, Dolanmaz D, Kalayci A. Intraosseous screw-supported upper molar distalization. *Angle Orthod* 2004; 74 (6): 838-850.

Glauser R, Sch€upbach P, Gottlow J. Periimplant soft tissue barrier at experimental one- piece mini-implants with different surface topography in humans: a light-microscopic overview and histometric analysis. *Clin. Implant Dent. Relat. Res*. 2005;7(1):44-51.

Greener E, Lauten Schlager E. 'Materials for Bioengineering Applications' In: Brown JHV, Jacobs JE and Stuart L (Eds): *Biomedical Engineering, Philadelphia,* FA Davis, 1971.

Grosgogeat B.: résistance à la corrosion et biocompatibilité des fils orthodontiques. *Orthodontie Française* 2002; 74: 115-121.

Guyonnet J, Escalassan R, Gregoire G. Electrogalvanisme buccal. *Encycl. Méd. Chir. Odontologie* 2008; 23-063-D-10.

Han M, Chung C, Choi H. A study on surface alteration of implant screws after function. *J. Korean Acad. Prosthodont*. 2002; 40 (3):275–86.

Hanning M. Transmission electron microscopy of early plaque formation on dental materi- als. *Eur. J. Oral. Sci*. 1999; 107: 55-64.

Heitz-Mayfield LJ. Peri-implant diseases: diagnosis and risk indicators. Proceedings from the 6th European Workshop on Periodontology. *J. Clin. Periodontol.* 2008; 35: 292-304.

Higuchi KW, Slack JM. The use of titanium fixtures for intraoral anchorage to facilitate orthodontic tooth movement. *Int. J. Oral. Maxillofac Implants*. 1991; 6 (3): 338-44.

House K, Sernetz F, Dymock D, Sandy J. R, Ireland A J. Corrosion of orthodontic appliances - should we care? *Am. J. Orthod. Dentofacial Orthop*. 2008;133: 584-92.

Kim. J, Ahn. S. Histomorphometric and mechanical analyses of the drill-free screw as orthodontic anchorage. *Am. J. Orthod. Dentofacial Orthop*. 2005; 128:190-4.

Kim HJ, Yun HS, Park HD, Kim DH, Park YC. Soft tissue and cortical-bone thickness at orthodontic implant sites. *Am. J. Orthod. Dentofacial Orthop*. 2006; 130 (2): 177–82.

Kraut RA, Hammer HS, Wheeler JJ. Use of endosteal implants as orthodontic anchorage. *Compendium*. 1988;9(10):796-7, 800-1.

Kuroda S, Sugawara Y, Deguchi T, Kyung HM, Takano-Yamamoto T. Clinical use of miniscrew implants as orthodontic anchorage: success rates and postoperative discomfort. *Am. J. Orthod. Dentofacial Orthop*. 2007; 131 (1):9-15.

Lijima M, Muguruma T, Brantley W, Okayama M. Torsional properties and microstructures of miniscrew implants. *Am. J. Orthod. Dentofacial Orthop*. 2008; 134 (3): 333.e1–6 [discussion 333–4].

Liliane S. Morais a,b, Glaucio G. Serra a,b, Carlos A. Muller c, Leonardo R. Titanium alloy mini-implants for orthodontic anchorage: Immediate loading and metal ion release. *Acta. Biomaterialia* 2007; 3 331-339.

Lin JC, Liou EJ, Yeh CL. Intrusion of overerupted maxillary molars with miniscrew anchorage. J. *Clin. Orthod.* 2006; 40 (6):378-383; quiz 358.

Lindhe J. Meyle J. Peri-implant diseases: Consensus Report of the Sixth European Workshop on Periodontology. Group D of European Workshop on Periodontology. *J. Clin. Periodontol.* 2008; 35: 282-285.

Massif. L, L. Frapier. Utilisation clinique des minivis en orthodontie. Encycl Méd Chir Odontologie/Orthopédie Dentofaciale, 2006; 23-492-A-17.

Matasa C.: attachment corrosion and its testing. *J. clinortho*d. 1995; 29 (1): 16-23.

Melsen B, CostaA. Immediate loading of implants used for orthodontic anchorage. *Clin. Orthod. Res.* 2000; 3: 23-8.

Melsen B, Lang NP. Biological reactions of alveolar bone to orthodontic loading of oral implants. *Clin. Oral Implants Res*. 2001; 12 (2):144-152.

Messer R,1 Tackas G, Mickalonis J, Brown Y. Corrosion of Machined Titanium Dental Implants Under Inflammatory Conditions. J Biomed Mater Res 2009; Part B: *Appl. Biomater*. 88B: 474-481.

Miyawaki S, Koyama I, Inoue M, Mishima K, Sugahara T, Takano-Yamamoto T. Factors associated with the stability of titanium screws placed in the posterior region for orthodontic anchorage. *Am. J. Orthod. Dentofacial Orthop*. 2003; 124 (4):373-378.

Moon IS, Berglundh T, Abrahamsson I, Linder E, Lindhe J. The barrier between the keratinized mucosa and the dental implant. An experimental study in the dog. *J. Clin. Periodontol*. 1999; 26 (10): 658–63.

Morais LS, Serra GG, Muller CA, Andrade LR, Palermo EFA, Elias CA, et al. Titanium alloy mini-implants for orthodontic anchorage: immediate loading and metal ion release. *Acta. Biomater* 2007; 3: 331–9.

Muster D, Vouillot JL, Dubruille JH. Biomatériaux, biomatériels et bioingénierie en chirurgie orale et maxillo-faciale. *Encycl. Méd. Chir. Stomatologie-Odontologie* 1999; 22-014-F- 10.

Naim S, Gregoire G. Importance de l'état de surface dans l'approche de la biocompatibilité d'un biomatériau. *J. Biomat. Dent.* 1998; 13: 89-104.

Nanci A, Wuest J.D, Peru L, Brunet P. Chemical modification of titanium surfaces for covalent attachment of biological molecules. *J. Biomed. Mater. Res,* 40, 324–335, 1998.

Odman J, Lekholm U, Jemt T. Osseointegrate implants as orthodontic anchorage in the treatment of partially edentuleous adult patients. *Eur. J. Orthod.* 1994; 16: 187-201.

Oshida Y, Sachdeva RC, Miyazaki S. Microanalytical characterization and surface mod- ification of TiNi orthodontic archwires. *Biomed. Mater. Eng.* 1992; 2 (2): 51-69.

Oyonarte. R, Pilliar. R. Peri-implant bone response to orthodontic loading: Part 1. A histomorphometric study of the effects of implant surface design. *Am. J. Orthod. Dentofacial Orthop.* 2005; 128: 173-81.

Oyonarte. R, Pilliar. R. Peri-implant bone response to orthodontic loading: Part 2. Implant surface geometry and its effect on regional bone remodelling. *Am. J. Orthod. Dentofacial Orthop.* 2005; 128: 182-9.

Park HS, Bae SM, Kyung HM, Sung JH. Micro-implant anchorage for treatment of skeletal Class I bialveolar protrusion. *J. Clin. Orthod.* 2001; 35 (7): 417-422.

Park JB, Lakes RS. 'Metallic Implant Materials' ln Biomaterials - an Introduction, and ed, *New York, Plenum Press,* 1992:75-115.

Patterson E, Johns R. Theoretical analysis of the fatigue life of fixture screws in osseointe- grated dental implants. *Int. J. Oral. Maxillofac Implants* 1992; 7: 26-34.

Pazzaglia UE, Minola C, Gualtieri G, Gualtieri, Riccardi C, Cecillani L. Metal ions in body fluids after arthroplasty. *Acta. Orthop. Scand.* 1986; 57: 415-418.

Philippart F, Philippart-Rochaix M. « Les minivis »: un concept d'ancrage orthodontique. *International Orthodontics* 2004; 2: 319-330.

Picard B.: Biocompatibilité des métaux dans le milieu buccal. *Actualités Odonto-Stomatologiques* 1984; 145: 147-157.

Polat-Ozsoy O, Arman-Ozcirpici A, Veziroglu F. Miniscrews for upper incisor intrusion. *Eur. J. Orthod.* 2009; 31 (4) : 412–6.

Rangert B, Langer B. Binding overload and implant fracture: a retrospective clinical analysis. *Int. J. Oral. Maxillofac Implants* 1995; 10: 326–34.

Renault H, Georges-Renault G, Pierrisnard L. Les implants: chirurgie et prothèse: Choix thérapeutique et stratégique. *Editions Cdp* 2008.

Richard G. salivary Streptococcus Mutans levels in patients before, during and after orthodontic treatment. *Am. J. orthod. Dentofacial orthop.* 1991; 100: 35- 37.

Riendeau. F. Ancrage orthodontique intra-osseux à l'aide d'implants palatins. *J. Dent Québec* 2003; 40: 293-296.

Roberts WE, Marshall KJ, Mozsari PG. Rigid endosseous implant utilized as anchorage to protract molars and close an atrophic extraction site. *Angle Orthodontist* 1990; 60: 135-52.

Schou S, Holmstrup P, Stoltze K, Hjørting-Hansen E, Fiehn NE and Skovgaard LT. Probing around implants and teeth with healthy or inflamed peri- implant mucosa/gingiva. A histologic comparison in cynomolgus monkeys. *Clin. Oral Implants Res.,* 2002; 13: 113-26.

Schliephake H, Reiss G. Metal release from titanium fixtures during placement in the mandible: an experimental study. *Int. J. Oral. Maxillofac Implants* 1993; 8: 502–11.

Sebbar M, Bourzgui F, Aazzab B, Elquars F. Anchorage miniscrews: a surface characterization study using optical microscopy. *Int. Orthod.* 2011; 9 (3): 325-38.

Sebbar M, Bourzgui F, Badre L, El Quars F. Anchorage miniscrews: a histologic study of peri-implant soft tissue. Int. Orthod. 2012; 10 (1): 85-95.

Simon M, Lagneau C, Moreno J, Lissac M. Corrosion resistance and biocompatibility of a new porous surface for titanium implants. *Eur. J. Oral. Sci.* 2005; 113: 537– 545.

Soulet. A. Histoire de l'ancrage absolu. *Rev. Orthop. Dent. Fac.* 2006; 40; 2:153-175.

Sugawara J, Daimaruya T, Umemori M, Nagasaka H, Takahashi I. Distal movement of mandibular molars in adult patients with the skeletal anchorage system. *Am. J. Orthod. Dentofacial Orthop.* 2004; 125 (2): 130-138.

Urban RM, Jacobs JJ, Gilbert JL, Galante JO. Migration of corrosion products, from modular hip prostheses. Particle microanalysis and histopathological findings. *J. Bone and Joint Surg.* 1994; 76A: 1345-1359.

Wennerberg A, Albrektsson T. suggested guidelines for the topographic evaluation of implantsurfaces. *Int. J. Oral. Maxillofac Implants* 2000; 15: 331-344.

Wiechmann D, Meyer U, Büchter A. Success rate of mini- and micro-implants used for orthodontic anchorage: a prospective clinical study. *Clin. Oral Implants Res.* 2007; 18 (2): 263-267.

Wirz J. Matériaux, technologies et systèmes nouveaux et éprouvés. *Rev. Mens Suisse Odontostomatol.* 1998; 108 (3):225-227.

Zitzmann, NU and Berglundh, T. Definition and prevalence of peri-implant diseases. Proceedings from the 6th European Workshop on Periodontology. *J. Clin. Periodontol.* 2008; 35: 286-291.

In: Soft Tissue
Editors: A. J. Chavez Ruiz et al.
ISBN 978-1-62257-363-9

Chapter IV

Connecting Tissue Injury, Temperature and Mechanical Properties

Wei-Hsuan Huang and Chee-Kong Chui [*]
Department of Mechanical Engineering,
National University of Singapore, Singapore

Abstract

Temperature related tissue injuries are often present in most hyperthermia treatments. Tissue temperature and its mechanical properties are closely related due to the physiological changes caused by high temperature. An increase in tissue temperature will result in a decrease in moisture content in tissue, and permanent cell necrosis when temperature exceeds a threshold. It is therefore necessary to review the connection between temperature, mechanical properties and injury during hyperthermia treatment. A full understanding between the tissue temperature and mechanical properties allow for possible injury assessment through methods for detecting mechanical properties change such as Magnetic Resonance Elastography (MRE) and vice versa. Many forms of hyperthermia treatment exist in clinical practices; Radio-frequency (RF) ablation, Microwave ablation, Laser ablation, Ultrasonic ablation and Cryoablation. This publication concentrates on thermal injury caused by RF ablation and its effects on liver tissue temperature and mechanical

[*] Email: mpecck@nus.edu.sg

properties. RF assisted methods have been widely used in the treatment for hepatocellular cancers, breast tumors and cardiology treatments. RF ablation works on the principle of a high frequency electric current which generates ionic agitation and frictional heating in the target tissue. Catheters used for RF ablation are often needle electrodes for high current density and can be found in two forms; monopolar or bipolar electrodes. Monopolar electrodes work on the principle of a single polarity electrode with a large grounding pad attached to patients while bipolar electrodes are electrode pairs with dual polarity hence do not require a grounding pad. The electric field lines that are induced from the electrode tip by the applied voltage causes an electric force on the charged ions within the electrolytic medium of the liver tissue. This induced force produces a motion that causes ions in the tissue to rub against the surrounding fluid medium, causing friction and thus frictional heating. Increase in tissue temperature due to RF ablation results in moisture loss and protein denaturalization. Moffitt et al. (2002) and Walsh Jr et al (1989) both reported differences in mechanical property between native and thermally damaged liver. In our experi-ments, observations were also made for ablation time, to be positively related to a change in tissue stiffness. Ablation time is a good approxi-mation for tissue temperature and hence a relationship can be established between tissue temperature and mechanical properties. Mechanical properties of tissue can be measured by a compression test rig in-vitro or Magnetic Resonance Elastography (MRE) in-vivo. Temperature of tissue sample can be measured by thermocouple for point measurements and thermal cameras for plane measurements. Degree of tissue injury is not only a function of temperature but also a function of time exposed to a critical temperature. Liver tumor necrosis occurs at 45oC when held for long duration (hours) while necrosis occurs within minutes when temperature is above 60°C (Taton 2008, Baldwin 2001). Hence, tissue injury has to be correlated to temperature and exposed time. The degree of injury can be quantified by means of optical and fluorescence characteristics (Lin 2003) or Optical Coherence Tomography (OCT) (Wierwille 2010). Tissue variation is a big hurdle in the relationship between tissue injury, tissue temperature and mechanical properties. Microstructure variation in liver tissue causes non-systematic temperature distribution due to the many tissue variables; electric conductivity, thermal conductivity, blood perfusion rate, density, etc., governed by Joule heating and bioheat transfer equation. Hence affects homogeneity of RF ablation lesions and mechanical properties. A novel method is required to handle tissue variation for better simulation results and correlation between temperature and mechanical properties. A stochastic model might be a good approach to account for the tissue variation, while nondestructive medical imaging methods such as CT or MRI can be a topographic tool for large vessel placements in correlation models.

1. Introduction

Hyperthermia therapies are commonly used for cancer treatment. These therapies involve an elevation in tissue temperature (or reduction in the case of cryo-ablation) to induce cell necrosis in cancerous tumors. Temperature related tissue injuries are the basic mechanism present in hyperthermia treatments. These methods are effective due to the cytotoxicity observed in cells above a threshold temperature. In addition, S-phase cells which are the most ionizing radiation resistant are most sensitive to hyperthermia (Craciunescu 1999). There are many methods for energy deposition in hyperthermia treatment; Ultrasound ablation, Laser ablation, Radiofrequency ablation and Microwave ablation, etc. This book chapter concentrates on Radio-Frequency (RF) ablation, which is one of the most widely used hyperthermia method. Tissue temperature distribution is an important study in understanding RF ablation. Finite Element method is often used to simulate temperature of tissue undergoing RF ablation. Tissue temperature can then be related to cell death and categorized into mass ablation, carbonization, water vaporization, protein denaturation and membrane dissociation (Thomsen 2009). In general, an increase in temperature over a threshold, results in a change in tissue cell structure or content, moisture loss and protein denaturalization. The change in structure leads to a change in mechanical properties due to skeletal changes in cells. Studies reported differences in mechanical property between native and thermally damaged liver. In our experiments, observations were also made for ablation time, to be positively related to a change in tissue stiffness. Ablation time is a good approximation for tissue temperature and relationship can be established between temperature and mechanical properties.

The correlation of tissue injury/death to its mechanical properties is an interesting subject for study. Tissue injuries are often quantified in the micro scale by observing structures such as cells or equivalent during necrosis. Optical and fluorescence characteristics of tissue, histochemical markers or Optical Coherence Tomography (OCT) are methods available for quantifying cell death (Lin 2003, Wierwille 2010). However, mechanical properties of tissue are observed in the macro level such as tissue level for most pragmatic purpose. Test rigs such as a compression machine, Magnetic Resonance Elastography (MRE) and ultrasound elastography are choices for quantifying mechanical properties both in-vivo and in-vitro. Relationship between tissue injury and tissue mechanical properties helps us to relate the effect of an alteration of cell in a micro level on its macro level equivalent. A study of structural changes in the micro level, such as the skeletal structure of cells and extracellular matrix are often less commonplace in clinical practice, but only for specific interest groups.

This book chapter discusses the relationship between hyperthermia, tissue temperature, tissue injury and mechanical properties. The second section introduces fundamentals of Radio-frequency Ablation such as the differences between methods of RFA and their applications. Third section discusses the thermal effects on tissue which involves biophysics, heat transfer and Finite Element models. In the fourth section the link between tissue injury and micro structure is briefly discussed. Mechanical properties changes due to RF ablation are covered in the fifth section with correlation studies reviewed from existing work. Lastly, the future of hyperthermia is discussed with statistical based modeling techniques to account for tissue variation.

2. Isothermal Heat Treatments–Radiofrequency Ablation

Many forms of hyperthermia treatment exist in clinical practices - Radiofrequency (RF) ablation, Microwave ablation, Laser ablation, Ultrasonic ablation and Cryoablation. This section concentrates on thermal injury caused by RF ablation and its effects on liver tissue temperature and mechanical properties. RF assisted methods have been widely used in the treatment for hepatocellular cancers, breast tumors and cardiology treatments. RF ablation works on the principle of a high frequency electric current which generates ionic agitation and frictional heating in the target tissue. The electric field induced by the applied voltage causes an electric force on the charged ions within the electrolytic medium of the liver tissue. This induced force produces a motion that causes ions in the tissue to rub against the surrounding fluid medium, causing friction and thus frictional heating. The increase in temperature leads to coagulative necrosis in tissue (Haemmerich 2003).

Catheters used for RF ablation are often needle electrodes for its high current density. The catheters can be found in two forms - monopolar or bipolar electrodes. Monopolar electrodes work on the principle of a single polarity electrode with a large grounding pad attached to patients. The current density is highest at the electrode tip-tissue interface where area of contact is small and decreases when current flows through the body and exits from the grounding pad. Monopolar catheters enable electrode design to be small and slim, hence suitable for percutaneous or minimally invasive procedures. However due to the small area of contact, treatment area is limited. A possible way to increase treatment area is an expandable prong design which consists of retractable electrodes.

Bipolar electrodes are electrode pairs with dual polarity for current flow (Figure 1). It does not require the grounding pad as required for monopolar catheters. Bipolar electrodes can be arranged into electrode systems with 2 or more electrodes for large treatment area. Due to the close distance between electrodes, there is higher current density at the electrode-tissue interfaces and thus a higher and faster area of treatment in comparison to monopolar catheters. Bipolar catheters can be used for open surgery or to be integrated into laparoscopic devices (Chang 2011).

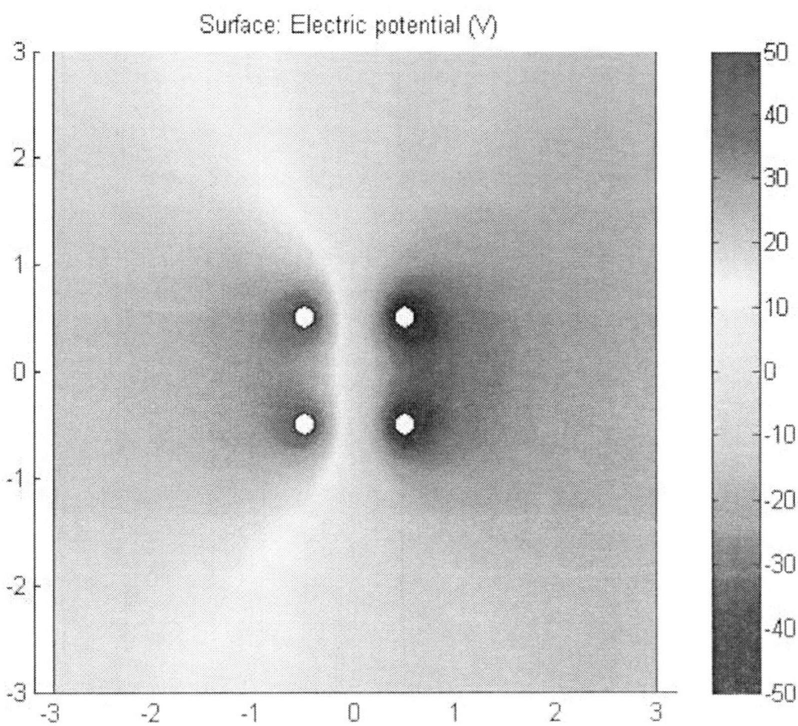

Figure 1. Bipolar electrode Electric Field Distribution.

Haemmerich et al (2001) investigated the differences between monopolar and bipolar Radio-frequency ablation with the use of a finite element model. It was concluded that the bipolar method creates larger lesions and is less dependent on local inhomogenities in liver tissue.

Lim et al (2010) studied the effect of different Radiofrequency waveform on tumor ablation with blood vessel heat sink effect. RF waveforms such as half-sine, half-square, half-exponential and damped sine wave were simulated. It was concluded that the damped sine waveform creates the smallest RF lesion in volume while the half-sine wave form is the most effective.

RF ablation is most commonly used to destroy tumorous cells as a form of direct treatment. Tumors are subjected to cytotoxic temperature and results in cell necrosis. However, there are other usages for RF ablation in medicine. Liver resection, also known as hepatectomy, is the gold standard for liver tumor treatment. It is desirable to minimize blood losses during liver resection procedure for best treatment survivability.

Dr Habib (Jiao 2006) pioneered a surgical procedure which uses RF ablation for hepatectomy. RF ablation was first performed on the desired line of resection to form a plane of coagulated tissue, followed by a manual resection with surgical scalpel. This reduces possible blood losses during resection and hence relieving usage of surgical maneuvers such as the Pringle maneuver (Milicevic 2008) which often results in results in ischemia-reperfusion hepatocellular injury. The technique can be performed by clinician whom is familiar with liver anatomy. The technique also results in reduction of the length of the anesthetic time and the operating time as it is much faster to achieve coagulation in normal liver tissue compared to tumors.

Another usage for RF ablation is in the treatment for large tumors (3~8cm in diameter). Although Hepatectomy remains the gold standard for liver tumor treatment, only a low percentage of patients are eligible for the procedure (Tranberg 2004). RF ablation serves as a good alternative treatment for liver tumors due to its low invasiveness, simplicity and cost effectiveness (Ni 2005).

Large tumor ablation is performed by overlapping zones of RF ablated tissue for full coverage of the tumor. In order to increase RF ablation area, many methods were developed such as saline injection (Livraghi 1997) for increased electrical conductivity, cooled electrodes to reduce charring (Goldberg 1996) and bipolar array to increase treatment zone area (McGahan 1996).

3. Thermal Effect on Tissue

Radio-frequency Ablation involves heat transfer in tissue which will be the main topic of discussion in this section. It is difficult to monitor actual temperature distribution in the tumor. Hence, it is suggested that modeling should be used for better understanding of the temperature distribution (Clegg 1993). Various works were done in modeling the RF ablation process with Penne's Bioheat Equation being the most commonly cited (Craciunescu 1998). While Penne's bioheat equation does not fully describe the full physical process of RF ablation, it is a good approximation especially for hyperthermia temperatures (Yang 2007).

It is due to the temperature dependence of many different physical parameters such as dielectric and thermal properties which is crucial for simulation. Harmmerich (2001) suggested that Penne's assumption of heat transfer between tissue and blood occurs is not an accurate description. Nevertheless, the model describes blood perfusion with good accuracy if no large vessels are near the area of concern. This limitation does not adversely affect the accuracy of Penne's model (Pennes 1948) in liver RF ablation as it is common to avoid the major vessel in the liver during surgery. It is also worth noting that variable such as conductivity; current density and blood perfusion do not change during ablation in Haemmerich's work and is assumed to be a constant in the model (6.4×10^{-3}).

A modified Pennes bioheat equation for RF ablation simulation:

$$\rho c \frac{\partial T}{\partial t} = \nabla \cdot k \nabla T + J \cdot E - \rho_{bl} c_{bl} \omega_{bl} (T - T_{bl})$$

where ρ is the density, c is the specific heat capacity of material, T is the temperature, k is the thermal conductivity, J is the current density, E is the electric field intensity, ρ_{bl} is the blood density, c_{bl} is the blood specific heat, ω_{bl} is the blood perfusion rate and T_{bl} is the blood temperature.

Finite Element Method (FEM) was used for simulation (Figure 2). The simulation incorporates the effect of Joule heating due to Electromagnetic energy which was not present in Penne's 1948 model. Chang and Nguyen attempted to model the radio frequency ablation process in soft tissue by means of a two dimensional finite element model (Chang 2004).

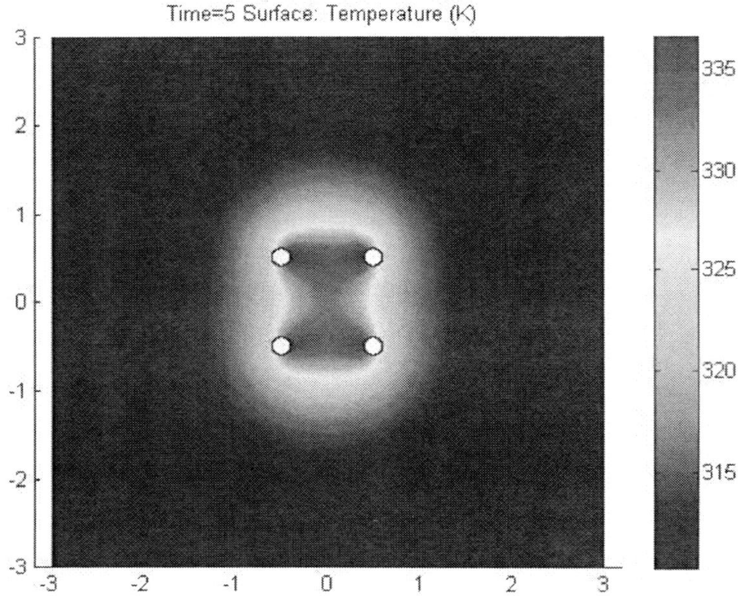

Figure 2. Finite Element Analysis of Bi-polar RF Ablation.

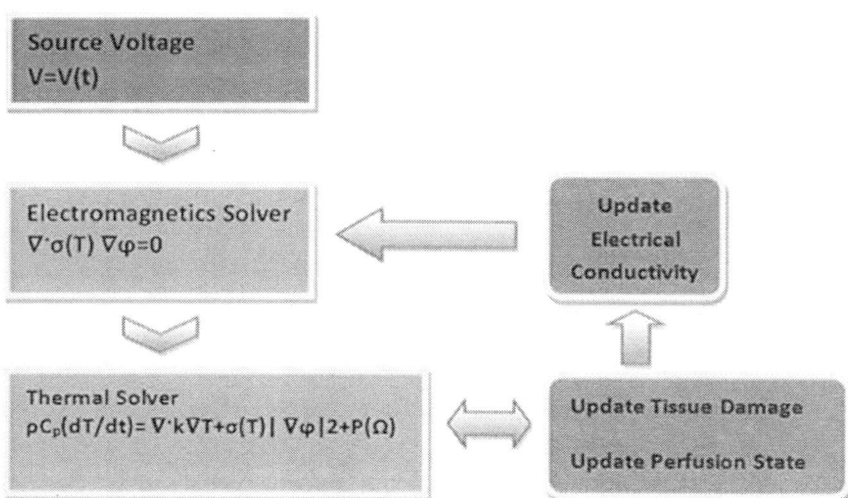

Figure 3. Illustration of Chang and Nguyen model (Chang 2004).

The model takes into account both the temperature and electrical conductivity dependence of the RFA process with respect to the tissue. The results was compared to lesion sizes which involves iso-temperature contour as its definition and concluded that temperature isotherms may not be the best representation for actual tissue damage pattern. The model (Figure 3) has a close loop, self updating structure consisting of the Specific Adsorption Rate (SAR) - the amount of energy absorbed by the tissue from the ablation needle, the Penne's bioheat equation for updating of tissue temperature, updating thermal conductivity of tissue and Arrhenius equation to update the tissue damage and perfusion related.

Tissue coagulation is assumed to occur when damage equation reaches a certain threshold (Ω=4.6) and that tissue coagulation is accompanied by the ceasing of perfusion. Once perfusion is stopped, the convective part of heat transfer due to perfusion is no longer valid, and the perfusion term is assumed to be zero. Ahmed et al (2008) used an established computer simulation model of radiofrequency ablation to characterize the combined effects of varying perfusion, and electrical and thermal conductivity on RF heating. The varying electrical and thermal conductivities are used to represent tissue, fats and saline injection. The different parameters were changed to model the effect of RF heating in different scenarios. It was concluded that greatest RF heating occurred when the ablation needle surrounded by tissue and with an outer layer of fats. However, the model does not account for coagulation of blood vessels and thus the stopping of perfusion. Solazzo et al (2005) studied the effect of a varying background electrical conductivity to RF heating effectiveness.

The team concluded that there is a strong relationship between background tissue and RF heating. Bellia et al (2008) proposed the simulation of Penne's bioheat equation with transmission line method (TLM) and showed good agreement with other numerical methods.Roper (2004) used an integral transformation to formulate a benchmark solution for bioheat equation. Comprison of the benchmark solution with numerical solution shows close matches. Yang et al (2007) proposed a new bioheat equation for microwave ablation which includes tissue water evaporation, diffusion, vapor diffusion and condensation due to the dominant of these physical processes when temperature reaches 100°C.

Arkin et al (1994) reviewed the different models proposed in modeling heat transfer in blood perfused tissue. The model aids in better predicting hyperthermia procedure which is relevant to the Radiofrequency Ablation technique we're studying. Due to the complex morphology of living tissues, hyperthermia modeling is often difficult and requires simplifying assumptions to be drawn. Penne's bioheat equation is inadequate in accounting for actual thermal equilibrium process between flowing blood and tissue. Penne's bioheat equation assumes that heat transfer occurs only through vessel walls and blood reaches tissue temperature immediately after entering the concerned vessel. Several techniques were reviewed for their strength and weaknesses. It was concluded that Pennes' model might still be the best practical approach. However, the main problem with bioheat transfer modeling remains the absence of measuring equipment capable of reliable evaluation of tissue properties and their variations at small scale. In addition, the model does not take into account denaturalization of the tissue causing structural changes and fluid exchanges when hyperthermia treatment is applied.

4. Mechanism of Cell Death

Tissue temperature is a direct cause of tissue injury which is quantifiable by cell death. All living cells are sensitive to temperature in certain degree. The result of thermal injury on different cellular structures and functions will ultimately determine whether the hyperthermia exposure results in reversible, partially reversibly or irreversible injury.

Plasma Membrane is the first contact with cell by conductive heating. When membrane is subjected to high temperature, it experiences phase changes into fluid form. Cytoskeleton is the structural proteins that form a filmentous network of microfilaments, microtubules and intermediate filaments. When subjected to hyperthermic treatments, the cytoskeleton loses its integrity and cells begin to round and fragment.

The effects of hyperthermia on nuclear structure and function may have relevance to the viability of myocytes subjected to hyperthermia. If marked nuclear disruption can be achieved in relevant temperature ranges. Wierwille et al (2010) examined RF ablation lesions with optical coherence tomography and noted significant differences between ablated and non-ablated tissue. Shrinking of muscle fibres and an increase in interstitial area (Figure 4) was observed for tissue which underwent RF ablation.

The ablated tissue has 31% less muscle to area ratio in relative. Larson et al (1996) examined the intraprostatic pathologic changes following accurately measured doses of transurethral microwave thermal energy in patients with benign prostatic hyperplasia.

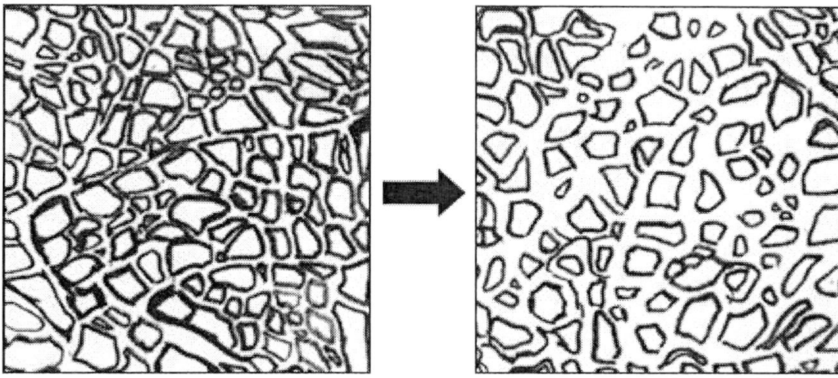

Figure 4. Changes in microstructure for tissue undergoing ablation. Increase in interstitial spacing and shrinkage in muscle fibre (Wierwille 2010).

Pathologic findings were similar in all cases, consisting of sharply circumscribed intraprostate thermal injury with uniform hemorrhagic necrosis and tissue devitalization without significant inflammation. Necrosis involved pure stromal nodules, mixed epithelial and stromal nodules, and predominately epithelial nodules. Mummified glands and stromal elements were noted in the areas of necrosis. Patchy acute and chronic inflammation was observed in the uninvolved prostate with a pattern suggesting mechanical disruption of the pathway for exit of secretions and consequent acinar rupture. Border between viable tissue and area of necrosis was sharply demarcated, extending no more than 1mm in thickness. This implied the tissue response to thermal energy was discrete rather than graduated. Thus, tissues exposed to a threshold thermal dose were devitalized, whereas tissues receiving lower thermal doses survived. Histopathologically demonstrable uniform thermoablation of a broad zone of obstructive prostate tissue can be achieved using an efficiently designed impedance matches transurethral microwave treatment catheter. Exposure of prostate tissue to temperatures higher than 45°C for approximately 1 hour is sufficient for the ablation process.

The rate and magnitude of cellular damage increases with temperature and time which is well represented by an Arrhenius Equation. Membrane bleb formation in human fibroblast is observed when exposed to supraphysiologic temperature. During RF ablation, the high electric potential on the thin membrane (5-10 nm) gives a high electric field, resulting in membrane dielectric breakdown and electroporation. Animal cells cannot survive the temperature and times of the temperature related to structural protein denaturalization. Therefore, if pathologic examination of the acute lesions shows thermal damage zones of characteristic structural protein denaturation such as collagen swelling, hyalinization and birefringence loss, all cells in those zones will be dead.

Tumor cell necrosis occurs at 45°C (Larson 1996) when held for long duration (hours) and within minutes when temperature is above 60°C (Taton 2008, Baldwin 2001). Supraphysiologic temperature due to Joule heating during RF ablation causes cell membrane rupture near a threshold temperature (Lee 1991). A high relevance paper by Thomsen (2009) described the mechanism of cell and tissue death due to thermal injury. While the paper was written for thermal injury instead of thermal therapy, they share many common grounds. Cell death was defined as chemical and/or genetic phenomena and events that either signal the inevitability of death or appear at or close to the point of no recovery. Trivial as it may seem, cell death due to hyperthermia is not an easy classification due to the presence of apoptosis. Apoptosis is a programmed cellular death triggered by cell signals and is a constructive process for cellular renewal. Hence, more efforts would be required to quantify cell deaths due to heat induced injury or the naturally occurring apoptosis.

There are primary and secondary thermal mechanisms for thermally induced cell deaths. Primary mechanisms are due to higher temperature and within targeted heated volume. Several mechanisms of primary effects causing cell death are tissue mass ablation, tissue caramelization and carbonization, water evaporation, extracellular/intracellular stromal protein denaturalization and thermal dissociation. Secondary thermal mechanisms are related to other physical, chemical or biological processes which eventually lead to cell death via triggering apoptosis. The secondary thermal mechanisms are not related to heat but are responses from the living tissue when subjected to physiological 'triggers'. Such 'triggers' include depletion of energy by stoppage of blood flow, production of reactive oxygen derived free radicals which causes mitochondrial dysfunction, changes in membrane chemical influxes and concentrations and release of cytokines causing immune host responses.

5. Mechanical Properties Due to Tissue Injury

Tissue injury or denaturalization results in a change in tissue modulus (Jiang 2007). Moffitt et al (2002) reported differences in mechanical properties between native liver and thermally damaged liver. It was concluded that the ultimate strength of native liver is higher than that of the thermally damaged liver. Walsh et al (1989) studied the effects of mechanical properties for guinea pig skin, bovine aorta, myocardium and liver on the efficiency of CO_2 laser ablation. It was concluded that ultimate tensile strength of tissue significantly affects the ablation efficiency. This draws an interesting insight as RF ablation and mechanical properties (tissue structure) are interrelated with RF ablation affecting mechanical properties and vice versa.

Kiss et al (2004) investigated the viscoelastic properties of normal and thermally damaged canine liver tissue which underwent different temperature treatment. Mechanical tests were done and the results fitted to the classic Kevin-Voigt model and Kelvin-Voigt Fractional Derivative model. Kelvin-Vogit fractional Derivative model was concluded to exhibit better fit to experiment data.

Obvious differences were observed between normal and thermally damaged tissue for the fit in the frequency domain, which exhibits viscoelastic properties. Huang et al (2011) studied the relationship between electrical impedance, tissue injury and mechanical properties. A model was built to examine how electrical impedance changes with ablation time and stress-strain relationship. Result was a 3D surface showing the correlation between the three parameters.

Compression testing experiment was conducted to study how mechanical property of the liver tissue changes with injury. Specimens of standard shape were obtained from freshly excised liver and subjected to RF ablation for different duration. The Arrhenius equation described in previous section justifies the principle of using ablation time to quantify tissue injury. The ablated or partially ablated samples were put into the test rig for compression test done up to 50% strain.

Experiment data were plotted and fitted with the Combined Energy Function by Chui et al (2004). The Combined Energy Function is a strain energy function that has been used to model the nonlinear stress-strain relationship of liver tissue. The Combined Energy Function equation:

$$\sigma = \left(2 + 2\varepsilon - \frac{2}{(1+\varepsilon)^2}\right)\left(\frac{C_1 C_2}{\left(6C_2 + 2 - 2C_2(1+\varepsilon)^2 - \frac{2C_2}{(1+\varepsilon)}\right)} + C_3\right)$$

The stress-strain data as well as the fitted curves are available in Figure 5. It is evident that sample exposed to a highest amount of RF ablation exhibits highest material stiffness during the initial stage of compression. Tissue stiffness eventually evens out between the samples at high strain. The reason could be due to the viscoelastic nature of soft tissue, where stiffness is a function of strain. As the strain increases, compacting of cells results in an increase in stiffness. Mechanical properties of tissue can be used as a measure of cell injury due to RF ablation in addition to other properties such as electrical impedance and optical properties. It is inevitable that the denaturalization of tissue caused by temperature results in tissue structure changes and hence changes in physical properties. Magnetic Resonance Elastography (MRE) is a choice for quantifying mechanical properties in-vivo. MRE is a noninvasive medical imaging technique which combines MRI images with propagating soundwaves into a map (elastogram). The elastogram shows the stiffness distribution of body tissue for the area of concern. The technique can be used to measure stiffness of tissue to differentiate between normal and ablated tissues.

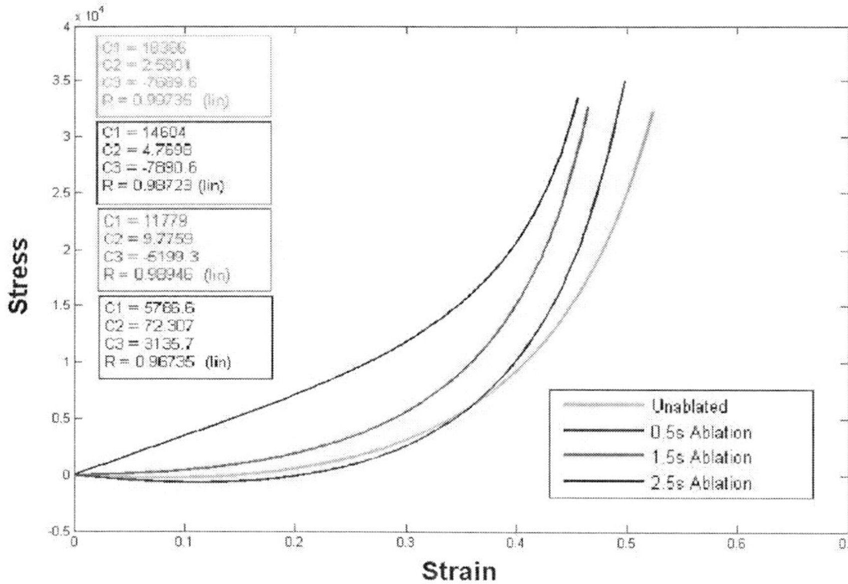

Figure 5. Compression Test results fitted with Combined Energy Function (Huang 2011).

Greenleaf et al (2007) developed a noninvasive technique to measure liver tissue stiffness by inducing ultrasonic radiation force to induce shear waves for propagation. The propagation speeds of the waves were measured as a function of frequency. The measured dispersion curve was then fitted to the Voigt model in determining tissue elastic and viscous moduli. Jiang et al (2007) explained the potential of using ultrasonic elasticity imaging to monitor tissue coagulations in-vivo and proposed a biomechanical model to study deformation-based strain imaging due to RF ablation. Rupert (2009) monitored Radiofrequency lesion with an ultrasound scanner for elastography. The strain image was then compared to actual pathologically examined tissue lesions and it was concluded that area of lesion in the elastography slightly underestimates the actual region.

6. Future of Hyperthermia

It was mentioned in previous section that a more complete model is required to accurately simulate the RF ablation process. Water evaporation, mass transport and vapor condensation are few of the many physical processes which really occur but are not accounted for in classical models (Jiang 2007). In addition, works on physical properties are needed for RF ablation simulation due to their temperature dependence. It is important to study how physical parameters such as dielectric and thermal properties vary with tissue injury and temperature. While mechanical properties are a function of temperature, Walsh (1989) concluded that it contributes to the effectiveness of hyperthermia treatments. The field of relating temperature, tissue injury and mechanical properties, tissue variation remains a hurdle in characterization of the properties.

Variations exist on the macro scale between patients, in anatomy of organs or vasculatures and on the micro scale, in cellular variations and bulk tissue properties. Various RF ablation simulation methods were reviewed in the earlier section. However, a common short-coming is the assumption of constant physical properties for all tissue samples. This assumption of constant physical properties in liver sample is inaccurate due to variation in micro structure and micro perfusion. In addition, liver tumors are angiogenic in nature thus altering perfusion state around the tumor. Variations in physical properties such as electrical conductivity, thermal conductivity, perfusion rate and density affect the final output of the simulation [19, 20] and should not be assumed to be identical. Statistical methods can be used to account for the variations in a statistical framework. Statistical methods were underway for the authors in developing a statistical based Finite Element method in simulating RF ablation in the liver tissue.

Stochastic Finite Element (SFE) method accepts a statistically distributed parameter values as input and produces output consists of a distributive simulation result. Tissue properties required for simulation are density, specific heat capacity, thermal conductivity and electrical conductivity. A normally distributed probability density curve for each physical parameter was constructed by taking the mean value from literature and standard deviation assigned to be 10% of the mean. Tissue blood perfusion properties such as blood temperature, blood volume and blood density are not randomized but assigned a value corresponding to the target tissue area perfusion state. For every RF ablation simulation, various physical parameter values were randomly selected from their individual probability density curve and used for the finite element simulation. It is evident that a peak is present in the output similar to the normally distributed parameter inputs (Figure 6). Drawing reference to statistical theory Central Limit Theorem, the close approximation of a normal distribution is viable when sample simulation size gets large.

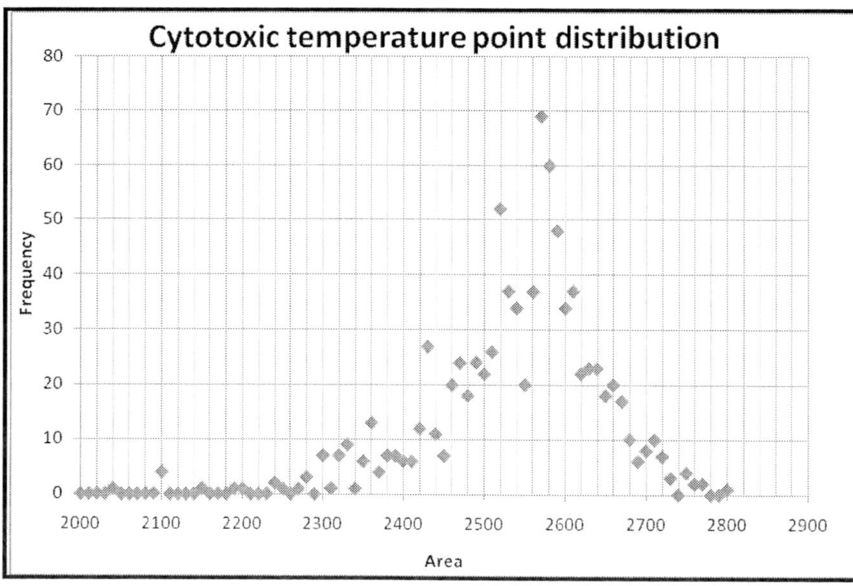

Figure 6. Output from Stochastic Finite Element Analysis.

The proposed method is hence statistical in nature and does not give a single solution. Similar approach can be used for modeling of tissue mechanical properties such as for parameters in Chui's combined energy function model or in the classic Voigt model.

Conclusion

In conclusion, relating tissue temperature, injury and mechanical properties will provide an insight into the science of hyperthermia treatment. While many work were done in simulating temperature distribution, observing histological changes and quantifying mechanical properties, there is a lack of work in relating these topics to fully understand how tissue react to temperature changes. In addition, statistical methods prove to be appropriate in tissue modeling due to innate tissue properties variation. The consideration of differences in properties will further enhance the accuracy of our current simulation and optimize the procedure and devices for best clinical effects.

References

Ahmed M, Liu Z, Humphries S, Goldberg SN, 2008. Computer modeling of the combined effects of perfusion, electrical conductivity, and thermal conductivity on tissue heating patterns in radiofrequency tumor ablation. *Int. J. Hyperthermia.* 24(7): 577-588.

Arkin H, Xu LX, Holmes KR, 1994. Recent Developments in Modeling Heat Transfer in Blood Perfused Tissue. *IEEE Transaction on Biomedical Engineering*, 41, 2, 97-107.

Baldwin S, Pelman A, Bert JL, 2001. A Heat Transfer Model of Thermal Balloon Endometrial Ablation. *Ann. Biomed. Eng.*, 29, 1009-1018.

Bellia SA, Saidane A, Benzohra M, Saiter JM, Hamou A, 2008. Dimensional soft tissue thermal injury analysis using transmission line matrix (TLM) method. *Int. J. Numer. Model,* 21, 531-549.

Chang IA and Nguyen UD, 2004. Thermal modeling of lesion growth with radiofrequency ablation devices. *BioMedical Engineering OnLine. BioMed Central.*

Chang S KY, Hlaing WW, Huang WH, Chui CK, 2011. Integrated ablation and division device for liver resection. *HPB,* 13(3).

Chui CK, Kobayashi E, Chen X, Hisada T, Sakuma I, 2004. Combined compression and elongation experiments and non-linear modeling of liver tissue for surgical simulation, *Medical and Biological Engineering and Computing*, 42, 787-798.

Clegg ST and Roemer RB, 1993. Reconstruction of Experimental Hyperthermia Temperature Distribution: Application of State and Parameter Estimation. *ASME Journal of Biomechanical Engineering*, 115, 380-388.

Craciunescu O, 1998. Influence of Blood Vessel Networks on Hyperthermia Induced Temperature Distributions. *UMI Dissertation Services*. PhD Thesis.

Craciunescu O, 1999. Influence of blood vessel networks on hyperthermia induced temperature. *UMI Microform* 9904030.

Goldberg SN, Gazelle GS, Solbiati L, Rittman WJ, Mueller PR, 1996. Radiofrequency tissue ablation: increased lesion diameter with a perfusion electrode. *Acad. Radiol.*, 3, 636-644.

Greenleaf JF and Chen S, 2007. Measurement of mechanical properties of homogeneous tissue with ultrasonically induced shear waves. *Medical Imaging,* 6513, 65130F-1.

Haemmerich D, Staelin T, Tungjitkusolmun S, Lee J, Mahvi DM, Webster JG, 2001. Hepatic Bipolar Radio-Frequency Ablation Between Separated Multiprong Electrodes. *IEEE Transactions on Biomedical Engineering.* Vol 48. 10.

Harmmerich D, Chachati L, Wright A, Mahvi D, Lee F,Webster JG, 2003. Hepatic Radiofrequency Ablation with Internally Cooled Probes: Effect of Coolant Temperature on Lesion Size. *IEEE Trans. On Biomedical Engineering,* 50, 4.

Huang WH, Chui CK, Kobayashi E, Teoh SH, Chang SKY, 2011. Multi-scale model for investigating the electrical properties and mechanical properties of liver tissue undergoing ablation. *Int. J. Comput. Assist. Radiol. Surg.,* 6(5), 601-607.

Jiang J, Varghese T, Chen Q, Hall TJ, Zagzebski JA, 2007. Finite Element Analysis of Tissue Deformation with a Radiofrequency Ablation Electrode for Strain Imaging. IEEE Transactions on Ultrasonics, *Ferroelectrics and Frequency Control,* 54, 2, 281-289.

Jiao LR, Navarra G, Weber JC, Havlic R, Nicholls J, Habib NA, 2006. Radio Frequency Assisted Liver Resection: The Habib's Technique. *Liver and Pancreatic Diseases Management,* 31-37. 2006 Springer.

Kiss MZ and T Varghese, 2004. Viscoelastic characterization of in vitro canine liver tissue. *IEEE International Ultrasonics, Ferroelectrics and Frequency Control Joint 50th Anniversary Conference*, 2086-2089.

Larson TR, Bostwick DG, Corica A, 1996. Temperature-correlated Histopathologic Changes Following Microwave Thermoablation of Obstructive Tissue in Patients with Benign Prostatic Hyperplasia. 1996 *Urology* 47 (4).

Lee RC, 1991. Physical Mechanisms of Tissue Injury in Electrical Trauma. *IEEE Transactions on Education,* 34, 3. 223-230.

Lin W, Buttemere C, Mahadevan-Jansen A, 2003. Effect of Thermal Damage on the In Vitro Optical and Fluorescence Characteristics of Liver Tissues. *IEEE Journal of Selected Topics in Quantum Electronics*, 9, 2, 162-170.

Lim D, Namgung B, Woo DG, Choi JS, Kim HS, Tack GR, 2010. Effect of Input Waveform Pattern and Large Blood Vessel Existence on Destruction of Liver Tumor using RF Ablation: Finite Element Analysis. *Journal of Biomechanical Engineering*, 132, 061003-1.

Livraghi T, Goldberg SN, Monti F, Bizzini A, Lazzaroni S, Meloni F, Pellicanò S, Solbiati L, Gazelle GS, 1997. Saline-enhanced radio-frequency tissue ablation in the treatment of liver metastases. *Radiology,* 202, 205-210.

McGahan JP, Gu WZ, Brock JM, Tesluk H, Jones CD, 1996. Hepatic ablation using bipolar radiofrequency electrocautery. Acad Radiol, 3, 418-422.

Milicevic M and Bulajic P, 2008. Radiofrequency-Assisted Liver Resection Does not induce severe liver damage. *World Journal of Surgery,* 32: 1901-1902.

Moffit T, Baker D, Kirkpatrick S, Prahl S, 2002. Mechanical Properties of Coagulated Albumin and Failure Mechanisms of Liver Repaired with the Use of an Argon Beam Coagulator with Albumin. *Journal of Biomedical Materials Research*, 63, 722-728.

Ni Y, Mulier S, Miao Y, Michel L, Marchal G, 2005. A review of the general aspects of radiofrequency ablation. *Abdominal Imaging*, 30, 381-400.

Pennes HH, 1948. Analysis of tissue and arterial blood temperatures in resting human forearm. *Journal of Applied Physiology*, 1:93-122.

Roper R and Jones M, 2004. Benchmark Solution for the Prediction of Temperature Distributions During Radiofrequency Ablation of Cardiac Tissue. *Journal of Biomedical Engineering,* 126, 519-522.

Rupert N, Bharat S, Dewall R, Andreano A, Brace C, Jiang J, Sampson L, Zagzebski JA, Lee F, Varghese T, 2009. In Vivo Ultrasound Electrode

Displacement Strain Imaging. *IEEE International Ultrasonics Symposium* Proceedings.

Solazzo SA, Liu Z, Lobo SM, Ahmed M, Hines-Peralta AU, Lenkinski RE, Goldberg SN, 2005. Radiofrequency Ablation : Importance of Background Tissue Electrical Conductivity – An Agar Phantom and Computer Modeling Study. *Radiology,* 236, 495-502.

Taton G, Rok T, Rokita E, 2008. Temperature Distribution Assessment during Radiofrequency Ablation. *IFMBE Proceedings* 22, 2672-2676.

Thomsen S, 2009. Targeted Thermal Injury: Mechanisms of Cell and Tissue Death. *Energy-based Treatment of Tissue and Assessment V,* Proc. Of SPIE Vol 7181.

Tranberg KG, 2004. Percutaneous Ablation of Liver tumours. *Best Practice and Research Clinical Gastroenterology,* 18, 1, 125-145.

Walsh JT and Deutsch TF, 1989. Pulsed CO2 Laser Ablation of Tissue: Effect of Mechanical Properties. *IEEE Transaction on Biomedical Engineering,* 36, 12, 1195-1201.

Wierwille J, McMillan A, Gullapalli R, Desai J, Chen Y, 2010. Quantitative Characterization of Radiofrequency Ablation Lesions in Tissue Using Optical Coherence Tomography. *IFMBE Proceedings* 32, 485-488.

Yang DS, Converse MC, Mahvi DM, Webster JG, 2007. Expanding the Bioheat Equation to Include Tissue Internal Water Evaporation During Heating. *IEEE TBME,* 54, 8, 1382-1388.

In: Soft Tissue
Editors: A. J. Chavez Ruiz et al.
ISBN 978-1-62257-363-9

Chapter V

Soft Tissue: Magnetic Resonance Imaging Findings of Myopathies

Daphne J. Theodorou**,
Stavroula J. Theodorou, and Yousuke Kakitsubata
[1]Department of Radiology, General Hospital of Ioannina and National Health Care System, Ioannina, Greece
[2]Department of Radiology, University of Ioannina School of Medicine
[3]Department of Radiology, Miyazaki Shakaihoken Hospital, Miyazaki, Japan

Abstract

Because the cause of musculoskeletal pain can be difficult to determine clinically in many cases, magnetic resonance imaging (MRI) is increasingly utilized to assess the anatomic location, extent and severity of several pathologic conditions offending muscle. MR imaging findings when correlated with clinical features and findings from other methods as electromyography may facilitate institution of correct diagnosis. Not infrequently, though, the presumptive diagnosis of skeletal muscle disease (myopathy) cannot be made on the basis of clinical- radiologic correlation; and, muscle biopsy is required to ensure diagnosis.Myopathy is suspected when patients complain that the involved muscle is painful

* D. J. Theodorou, MD, PhD, Email: rjtheodorou@hotmail.com.

and tender, experience difficulty performing tasks that require muscle strength, or develop various systemic manifestations as skin rash or respiratory problems. Infectious, inflammatory, traumatic, neurologic, neoplastic and iatrogenic conditions can cause abnormal signal intensity at MR imaging. Although diverse, some diseases have similar MR imaging appearances, whereas others present distinct patterns of signal intensity abnormality.

In general, alterations in muscle signal intensity fall into one of three cardinal patterns: muscle edema, fatty infiltration, and mass lesion. Because some of the muscular disorders, but not all, may require medical or surgical treatment institution of early diagnosis is important.

This chapter will review and illustrate the spectrum of MRI appearances in several primary and systemic disorders affecting muscle, both common and uncommon.We believe this work provides a collective —yet succinct and useful guide to a wide array of myopathies.

Keywords: Soft tissue, muscle diseases, MR imaging, skeletal muscle; myopathies, myositis, infection, muscle injuries, abscess

Introduction

Skeletal muscle abnormalities are commonly seen in orthopaedic, neurology or internal medicine practices, and share a wide variety of causes, treatments, and prognoses. Because patients with these conditions present with vague symptoms of myalgia, weakness, fatigue, and disability the abnormalities are often initially overlooked or even underestimated as a source of pathology [1, 2]. Furthermore, clinical assessment of the integrity and performance of skeletal muscle can be problematic, owing to the complex compartmental anatomy and several anatomic variations in muscle [3].

The diagnosis of muscle disease (myopathy) has typically relied on clinical examination, coupled with histological analysis of a muscle biopsy specimen in complex cases that may be obscure clinically. Early recognition of abnormalities is critical to implementing an appropriate management regimen that facilitates prompt and safe return to function and activity, however.

Due to the relatively nonspecific clinical presentation of primary and systemic disorders affecting skeletal muscles, imaging plays a key role in establishing the correct diagnosis. Radiography allows for evaluation of certain muscle derangements (i.e., infection, heterotopic ossification), but is limited by relatively poor sensitivity and lack of anatomic detail [4, 5].

CT facilitates the diagnosis of conditions similar to those detected by radiography in a cross-sectional display, but it provides limited contrast resolution for muscle. MRI has emerged as the advanced imaging method of choice for skeletal muscle, providing excellent soft tissue contrast resolution and multiplanar tomographic display.

Although many of the disorders affecting muscle may manifest with nonspecific imaging signs, MRI allows detection and characterization of these lesions that helps formulate a reasonable diagnosis. In addition, MRI may enable accomplishment of a limited differential diagnosis. Furthermore, MRI can depict selective abnormality within individual muscles that may be challenging to detect clinically because of the presence of unaffected synergistic muscles [6].

In this book chapter, we present the MRI findings seen with a wide array of primary and systemic neuromuscular and orthopaedic disorders that can aid the clinician when assessing the cause of pain and dysfunction in muscle. Although this work is not thought of as an exhaustive presentation of muscular pathology, we aim at presenting a concise, helpful and practical imaging review of the basic MRI findings associated with many common and uncommon musculoskeletal disease processes.

MRI Protocol

Many MRI protocols have been implemented for imaging muscle derangements. The simplified MRI protocol presented in this work is used at our institution borne out by our experience in evaluating suspected muscle pathology by a 1.5-T MR unit.

The patient is comfortably placed in the supine position to avoid pain, motion, and compression of different muscle groups. Occasionally, a marker (i.e., a nitroglycerin capsule) is used to point out the exact source of pain. Coronal and axial spin echo T1-weighted (TR/TE, 650-800/15-20) and fast spin echo T2-weighted (TR/TE, 3300-4550/90-140) sequences with fat suppression are performed. Alternative to the fat-suppressed T2-weighted sequence is a STIR (3000-3665/15-35, TI= 150 msec) sequence.

Images in a sagittal plane are occasionally acquired to match individual demands, and intravenous administration of gadolinium-containing contrast material is advised as appropriate.

Pathophysiology

In anatomy terms, muscle fiber comprises the basic structural element of skeletal muscle. The architecture and integrity of fibers in muscle is directly related to the **muscle's** function and mechanical behavior. Normal skeletal muscle function is dependent on intact muscle fibers, normal innervation, and sufficient blood flow. The application of abnormal mechanical stresses on muscle, as well as certain neurogenic disease processes causing neuropathic muscle dysfunction, several neuromuscular junction diseases, and different types of myopathies (i.e., metabolic, congenital) are all associated with net damage to the muscle cells, having variable effects on strength or motion [1, 2, 6]. Injury to the muscle-tendon-bone unit, which represents the structurally weakest portion of the muscle where muscle fibers join the tendon, also known as the myotendinous junction, is common and can vary by age. For instance, muscle injuries are more common in the young and tendon tears are more common in the elderly.

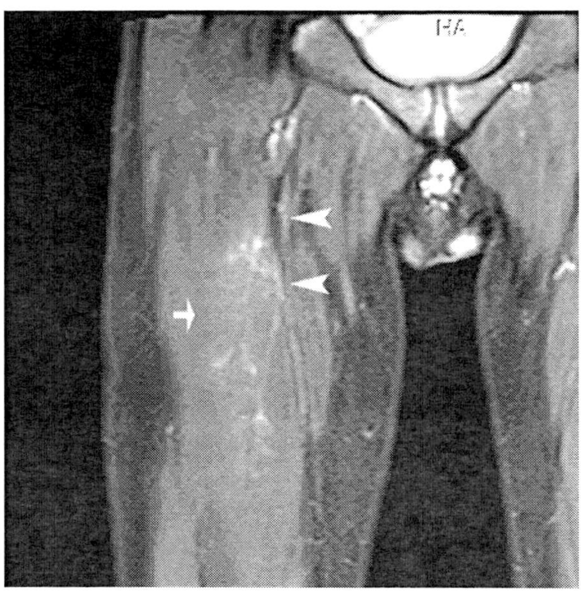

Figure 1. A 10-year-old boy who sustained a low-grade (Grade 1) strain in the rectus femoris muscle, 4 days after an injury that occurred while playing basketball. Coronal STIR MR image shows hyperintense signal (arrowheads) in rectus femoris surrounding thickened myotendinous junction and tracking along the muscle fascicles, in a feathery pattern (arrow).

Biomechanical and histopathology analyses have shown that skeletal muscle responds to various infinite insults with only a limited number of nonspecific biologic responses (i.e., edema, atrophy, fibrosis). For example, in physical trauma the healing process represents repair in the form of a fibrous scar rather than true regeneration of the injured muscle. Indeed, a wide array of primary and systemic disease processes affecting muscle can present with similar gross pathologic features.

MR imaging plays an important role in detecting alterations in muscle morphology and signal intensity characteristics associated with many disorders. Because the MR imaging findings of muscle disease may reflect gross underlying pathology rather than provide specific features for imaging diagnosis, inclusive differential diagnosis may eventually need to be entertained.

To facilitate the challenging diagnostic process, MR imaging and associated pathologic changes of parenchymal alterations in skeletal muscle are systematically classified into three major patterns based practically on the presence of edema, fatty infiltration, or a mass as presented below [1, 7].

Major Patterns of Muscle Involvement

A) Muscle Edema Pattern

Acute or recent muscle insult is characterized most commonly by edema, vascular engorgement, and inflammatory cellular infiltration [2]. As a rule of thumb, these nonspecific pathologic changes correspond to areas of low to intermediate signal intensity on T1-weighted images and high signal intensity on T2-weighted and inversion recovery images.

Many conditions reflecting a recent insult or a biologically active process can produce similar changes in signal intensity including traumatic injury (i.e., strain, contusion); muscular exertion (i.e., Delayed Onset Muscle Soreness, DOMS); rhabdomyolysis; vascular insults (i.e., compartment syndrome, diabetic infarction); myositis (i.e., autoimmune, idiopathic, infectious, sarcoid myopathy); early myositis ossificans; subacute denervation; and radiation therapy [1, 4, 5, 8-10]. Representative cases are illustrated herein (Figures 1-12).

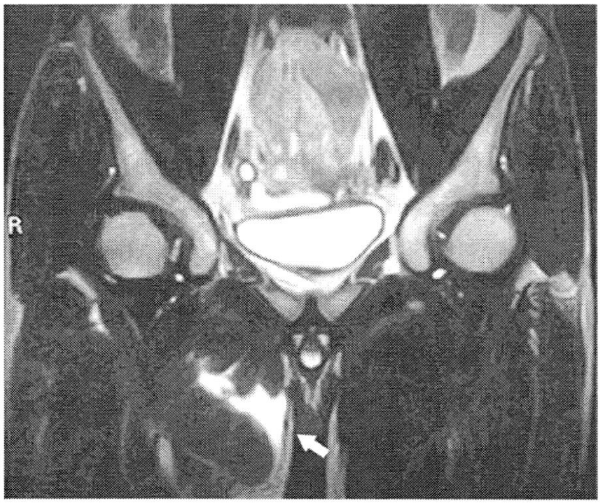

Figure 2. Adductor longus tear in a 16-year-old young man, 2 days after a bowling injury. Coronal T2-weighted MR image of anterior thigh demonstrates fluid signal (arrow) collecting at the site of complete fiber disruption, indicating a high-grade (Grade 3) injury.

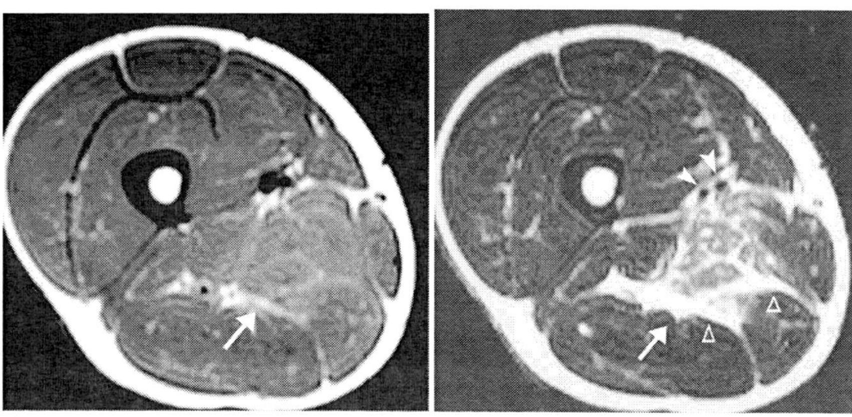

(a) (b)

Figure 3. Adductor magnus muscle contusion in a 24-year-old male hockey player, 2 weeks after a direct blow to the thigh. (a) Axial T1-weighted image of right midthigh shows only minimal signal alteration (arrow) in the adductor magnus muscle representing subacute hemorrhage into muscle. (b) Axial T2-weighted MR image shows abnormal high signal intensity within the substance of the adductor magnus muscle (arrow) due to edema and hemorrhage, which also outlines adjacent femoral neurovascular structures (arrowheads). Perifascial edema (open arrowheads) is also seen.

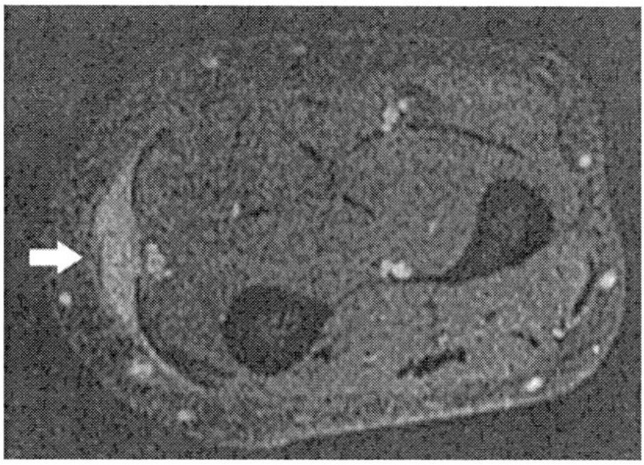

Figure 4. Delayed-onset muscle soreness (DOMS) in a 24-year-old female hairdresser, one day after intense manual labour. Axial STIR image demonstrates increased signal intensity (arrow) in the extensor carpi radialis brevis muscle. Soreness subsided within one week of rest.

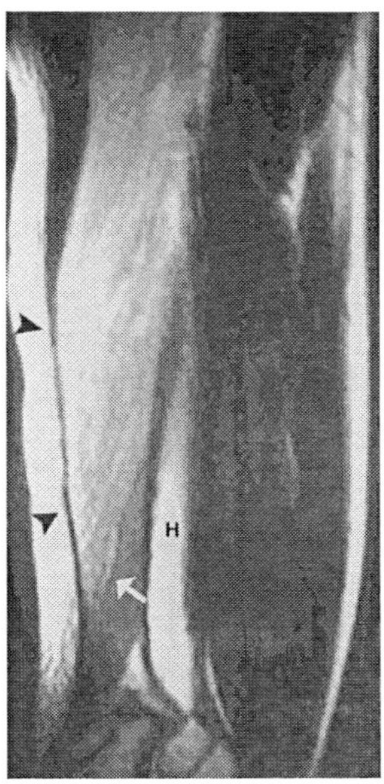

Figure 5. Rhabdomyolysis in a 13-year-old boy with gradual onset of pain in his arms after an intense weight-lifting workout. Sagittal T2-weighted MR image through the upper arm displays diffuse increased signal intensity in triceps brachii muscle (arrowheads). Note that edema-like signal tracks along muscle fascicles assuming characteristic feathery appearance (arrow) that reflects architecture of muscle. Associated myoglobinuria confirmed diagnosis of exertional rhabdomyolysis of left triceps brachii. H= humerus.

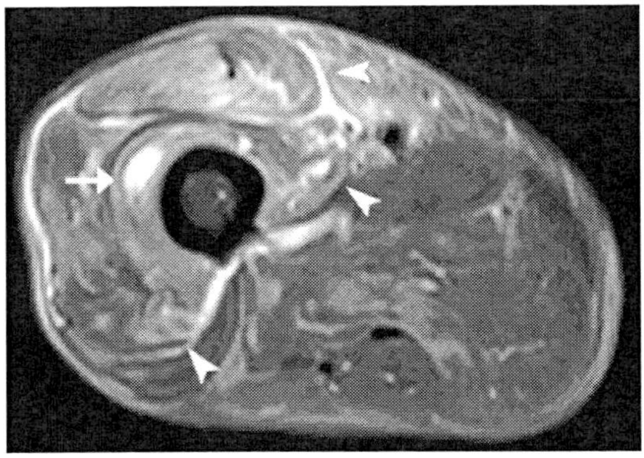

Figure 6. Acute compartment syndrome in a 46-year-old man who developed severe proximal thigh pain one day after injury in a motor vehicle accident. Axial STIR image shows diffuse hyperintensity of the anterior compartment muscles (arrowheads), but no osseous abnormalities. A small haematoma (arrow) is present in the vastus intermedius muscle. Compartment pressures were subsequently measured and confirmed the diagnosis of compartment syndrome.

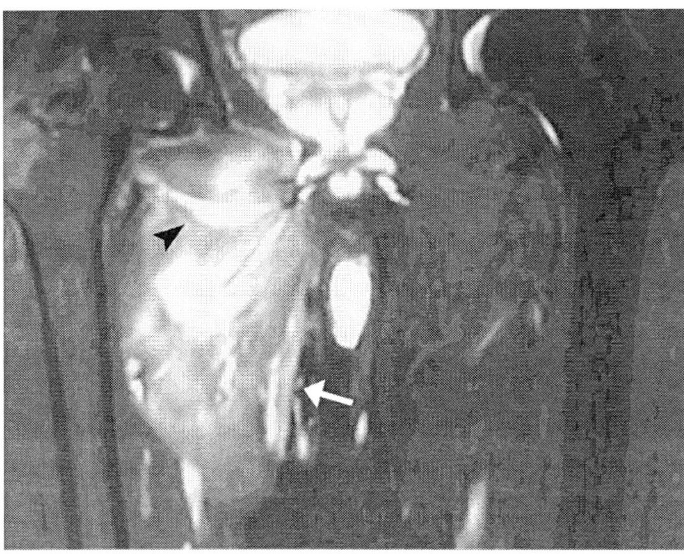

Figure 7. A 52-year-old poorly controlled diabetic man presenting with sudden onset of severe pain in the proximal thigh and buttocks, and muscle infarction. Coronal, fat-suppressed T2-weighted MR image shows extensive intramuscular edema in the anteromedial thigh involving the obturator externus, pectineus, and the adductor brevis and longus muscles (arrow). A small collection of fluid (arrowhead) is noted between the obturator externus and pectineus muscles.

B) Fatty Infiltration Pattern

Chronic muscle insult results in abnormal fatty infiltration of muscle characterized by the presence of fat signal intensity on both T1-weighted and T2-weighted images. Associated muscle atrophy is common. Severe muscle injury or chronic musculotendinous injury (i.e., tendon tear); chronic disuse; chronic denervation; myopathy (muscular dystrophy, mitochondrial myopathy,); lipomatous lesions; and corticosteroids are among the conditions associated with fatty infiltration atrophy [1, 2, 6, 7, 11-13]. Selected cases are illustrated accordingly (Figures 13-19).

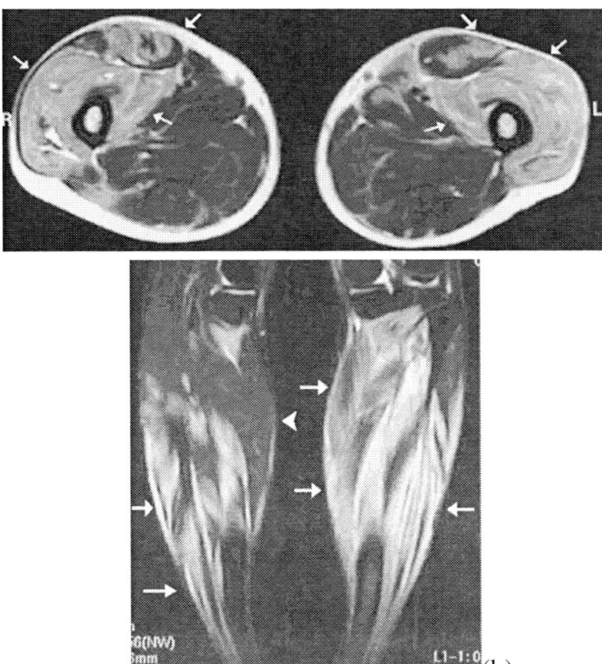

(a)

(b)

Figure 8. Polymyositis in a 26-year-old woman who presented with bilateral lower extremity pain and muscle weakness. (a) Axial T2-weighted MR image of the thighs shows abnormal, widespread feathery edema in the vastus lateralis, intermedius, medialis, and the rectus femoris muscles (arrows). Note the preservation of normal muscle architecture. T1-weighted imaging (not shown) did not display signal alteration or atrophy in affected muscles, or otherwise contribute to diagnosis in this case. (b) Coronal fat-suppressed T2-weighted MR image of both legs also shows extensive edema signal in muscles of the calf (arrows). Medial head of right gastrocnemius muscle appears spared (arrowhead).

These pathologic changes result in muscle contraction and stiffness, which in turn, alter biomechanics and predispose weakened muscle to further injury during weight bearing and muscle exertion.

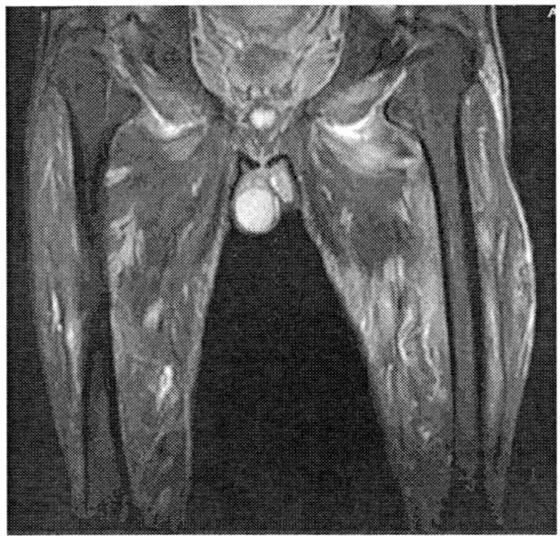

Figure 9. Idiopathic myositis in a 57-year-old man with sudden onset of muscle weakness, tenderness, and inability to walk. Coronal STIR MR image through the pelvis, hips and the thighs shows diffuse edema of the pelvic and thigh muscles. Muscle biopsy disclosed "**nonspecific**" myositis. The symptoms resolved over a six-month period, and the patient was able to resume full physical activity.

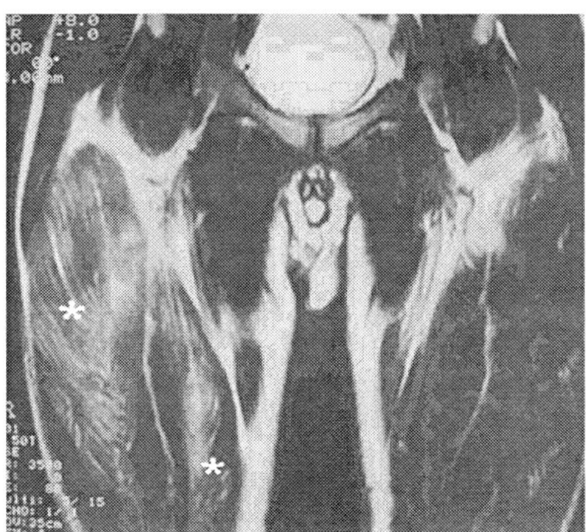

Figure 10. Infectious myositis manifest as edema in the right quadriceps muscles (asterisks) of a 34-year-old HIV-positive man, who presented with a swollen painful thigh and fever. Notably, there is no abscess formation that would have caused a mass-like appearance on MR images.

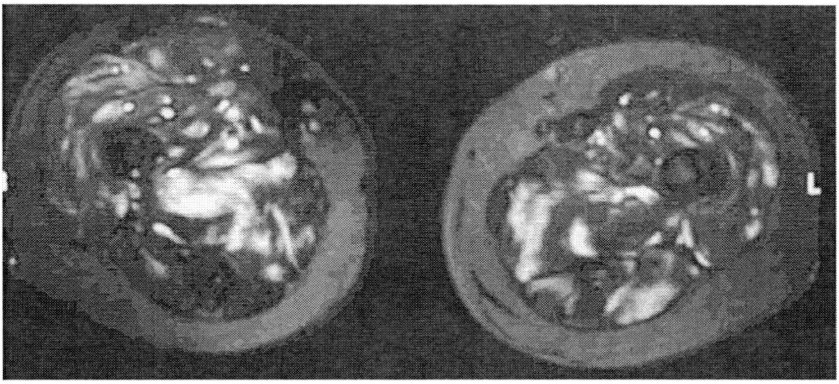

Figure 11. Sarcoid myopathy in a 52-year-old woman presenting with muscle weakness, myalgias, and elevated muscle enzyme levels. Axial fat suppressed T2-weighted MR image through the thighs shows extensive, high signal intensity edematous changes involving all muscle compartments, in both thighs. Biopsy revealed noncaseating granulomatous, lymphocytic infiltration, and muscle necrosis.

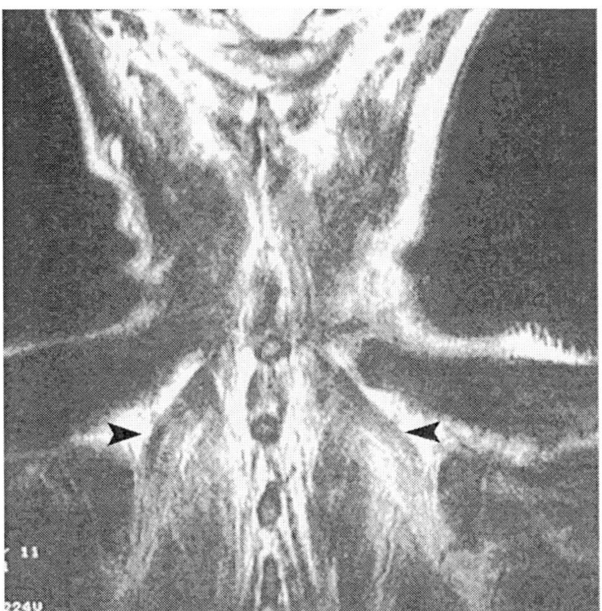

Figure 12. A 53-year-old woman with muscle edema after radiation therapy for lung cancer. Coronal T2-weighted MR image shows edematous and enlarged paraspinal muscles (arrowheads), in radiation field.

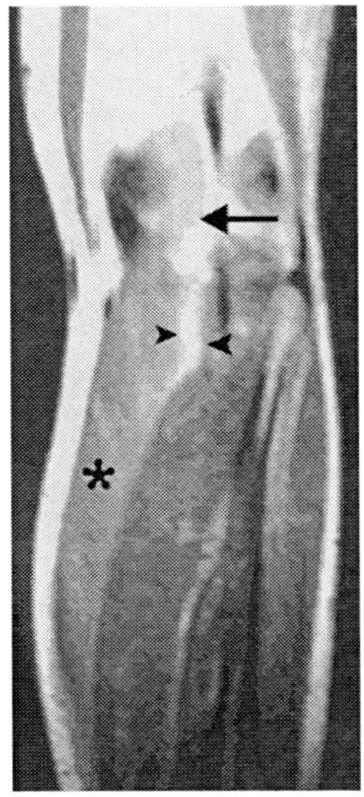

Figure 13. Old partial disruption of the proximal gastrocnemius muscle fibers at the musculotendinous junction (MTJ) region, in a 27-year-old man who was injured while running a marathon. Coronal T1-weighted MR image of the calf shows increased signal intensity within the medial gastrocnemius muscle (asterisk) and high signal intensity adjacent to the aponeurosis owing to abnormal deposition of fat (arrowhead). Findings of chronic partial tear of the proximal gastrocnemius fibers at the MTJ region (arrow) are seen.

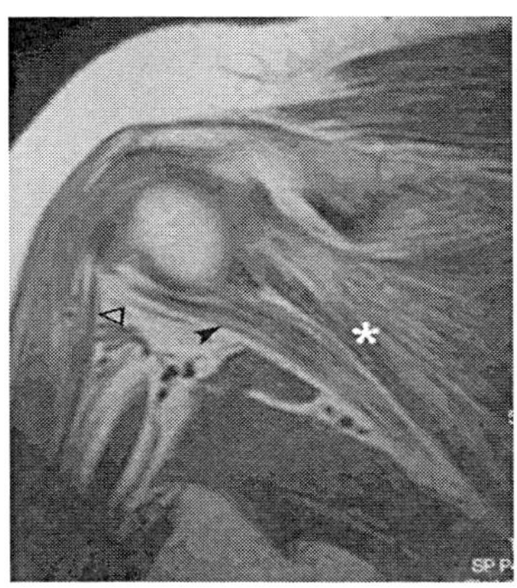

Figure 14. Chronic disuse in a 58-year-old woman with recurrent dislocations of the shoulder that resulted in limited use of her right arm. Coronal T1-weighted MR image shows extensive fatty infiltration of the infraspinatus (asterisk), teres minor (arrowhead), and deltoid (open arrowhead) muscles due to disuse.

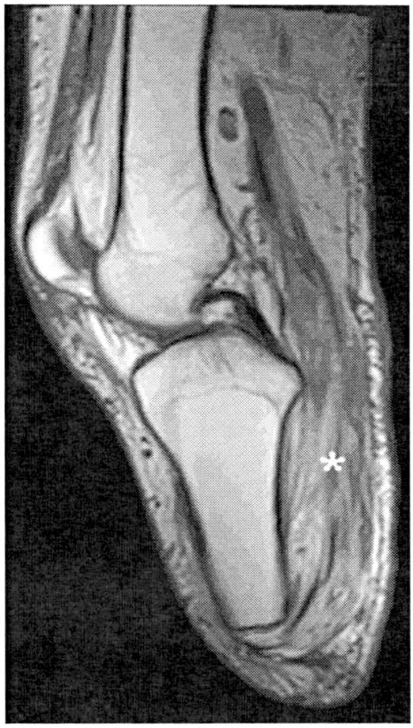

Figure 15. Chronic disuse in a 43-year-old man who had below-knee amputation after a motorcycle accident 12 years earlier. Sagittal T1-weighted MR image shows increased signal indicating fatty infiltration of gastrocnemius and popliteus (asterisk) muscles.

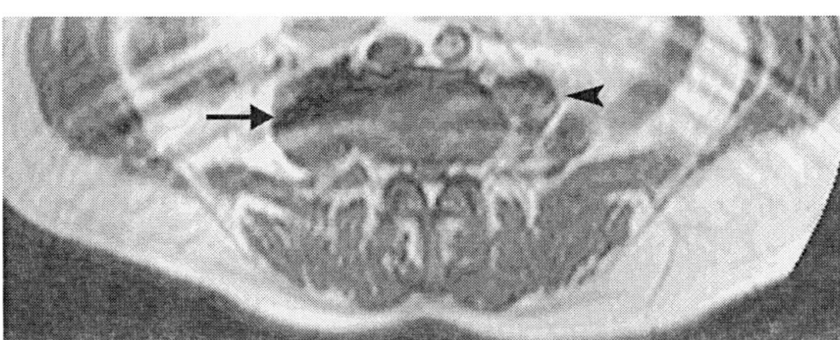

Figure 16. Chronic denervation of left psoas muscle in a 56-year-old man with poliomyelitis at age 3. Axial T1-weighted MR image shows fatty infiltration of left psoas (arrowhead) with marked decrease in muscle volume. Contralateral psoas muscle appears hypertrophic (arrow).

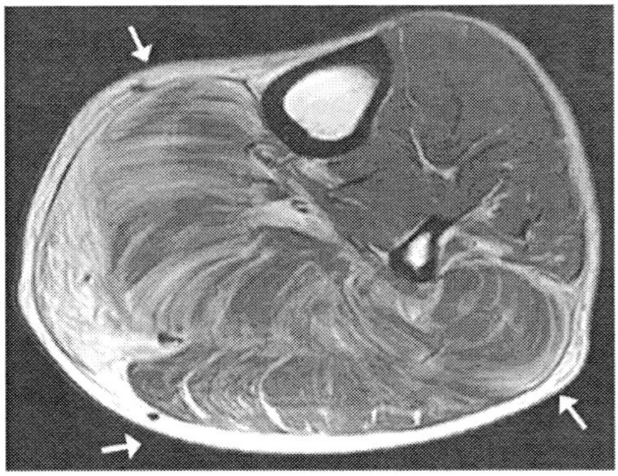

Figure 17. Charcot-Marie-Tooth disease (hereditary motosensory neuropathy) in a 58-year-old man with left leg swelling and weakness. Axial T1-weighted MR image of left calf shows diffuse abnormal high signal intensity in enlarged soleus and gastrocnemius muscles (arrows), reflecting gross fatty replacement.

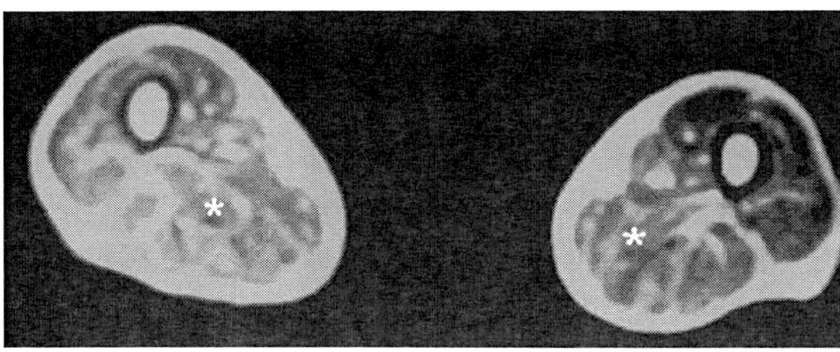

Figure 18. Mitochondrial myopathy in a middle-aged man. An axial T1-weighted MR image of the thighs shows almost symmetrical, fatty infiltration and atrophy of the quadriceps muscles (asteriks).

C) Mass Lesion Pattern

The mass lesion pattern refers to the presence of a space-occupying lesion in muscle. The MRI characteristics of lesions producing a mass effect are variable and typically different than those of normal muscle on all pulse sequences. Infection (i.e., pyomyositis, abscess, parasitic infection); traumatic injury (i.e., hematoma); myositis ossificans; myonecrosis; muscular sarcoidosis; and neoplasms (i.e., lipoma, liposarcoma, leiomyosarcoma) are all associated with an intramuscular mass lesion [4, 5, 9, 10, 14-16] (Figures 20-26). MRI provides characterization of mass composition that may reveal clues to the nature of a given lesion.

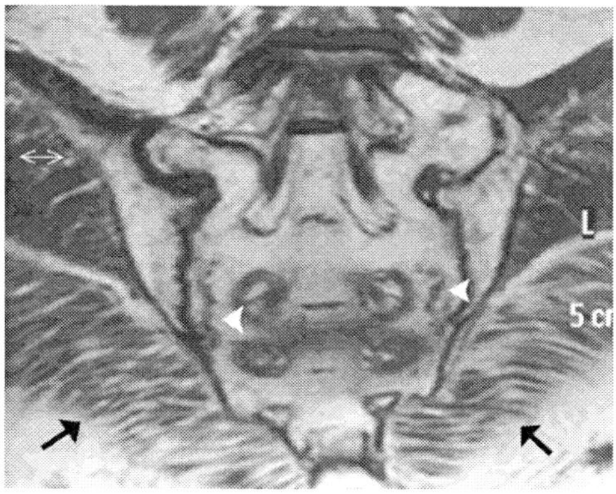

Figure 19. Fatty infiltration in a 52-year-old woman receiving long-term corticosteroids for rheumatoid arthritis. Coronal T1-weighted MR image shows prominent fatty infiltration and atrophy of gluteal muscles (arrows). Bilateral, steroid-induced osteoporotic sacral fractures are apparent (arrowheads).

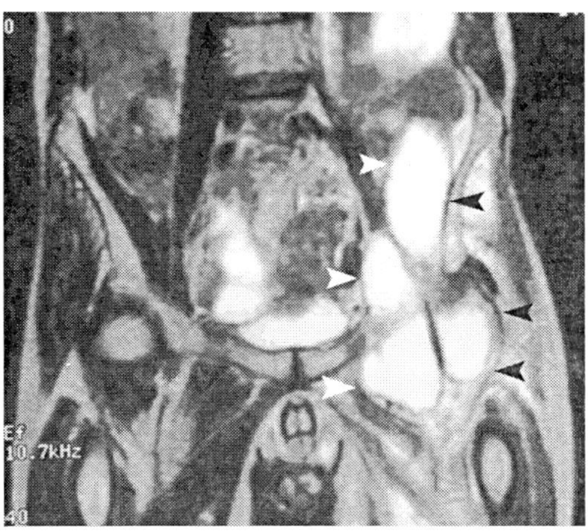

Figure 20. Pyomyositis with abscess formation in a 59-year-old man who sustained direct trauma to the hip and presented with pain of the left thigh, fever, and malaise.Coronal T2-weighted MR image shows multiple, large, sausage-like high signal intensity abscesses (arrowheads) adjacent to the wing of ilium and anterior to the hip joint on left side. Cultures of the abscess material retrieved Staphylococcus aureus.

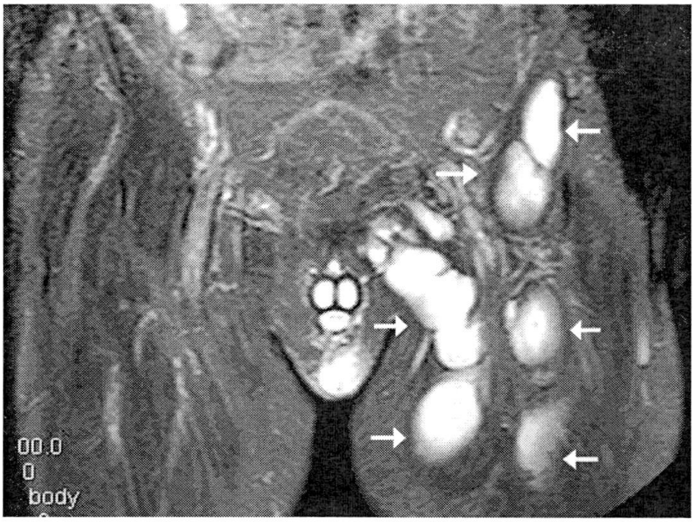

Figure 21. Muscular echinococcosis in a 46-year-old farmer with painful swelling of musculature in the proximal thigh and hip. Coronal fat-suppressed T2-weighted MR image shows large, loculated hyperintense parasitic cysts (arrows) in muscles of left thigh and hip.

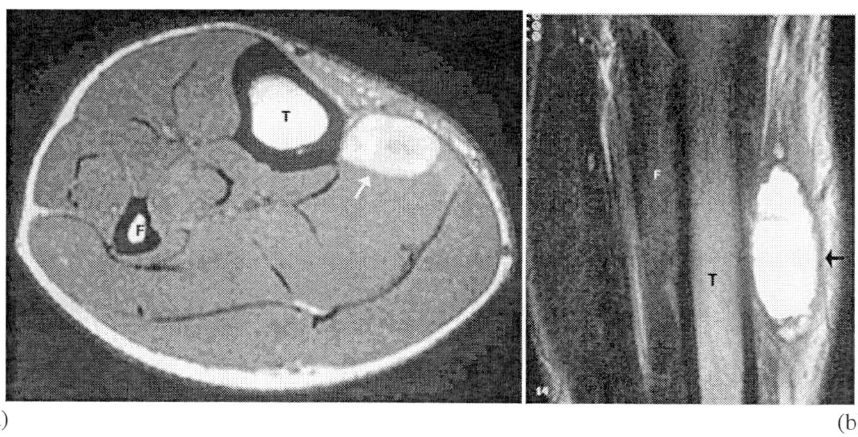

Figure 22. Intramuscular haematoma caused by a direct blow to the right calf in a 15-year-old boy during a hockey game one week earlier. Axial T1-weighted MR image (a) and coronal T2-weighted MR image (b) show a subacute haematoma of homogeneous high signal intensity in the gastrocnemius muscle (arrow). T= tibia, F= fibula.

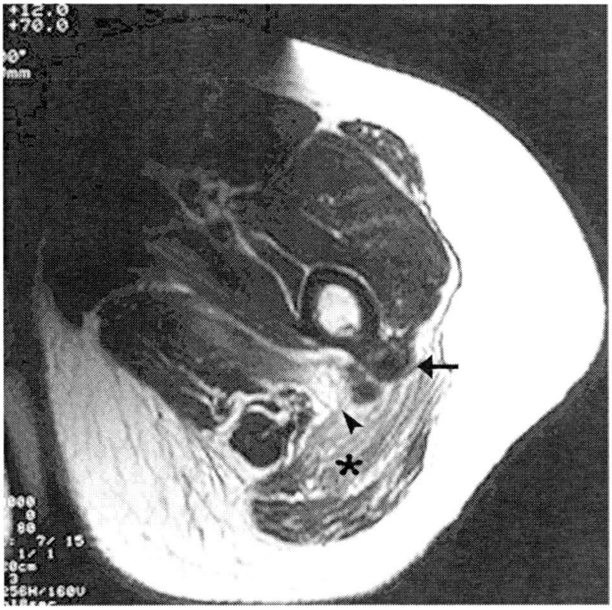

Figure 23. Myositis ossificans presenting as a painful and palpable mass in the left quadriceps musculature. T2-weighted MR image shows mature ossifying lesion of low signal intensity adjacent to the proximal femur (arrow), and a high signal intensity mass in the surrounding soft tissue (arrowhead). Abnormal high signal intensity corresponding to edema is seen infiltrating the gluteus maximus muscle (asterisk). On excision, the mass in the gluteus maximus was found to be immature myositis ossificans, while mature bone was retrieved from lesion in the quadriceps muscles.

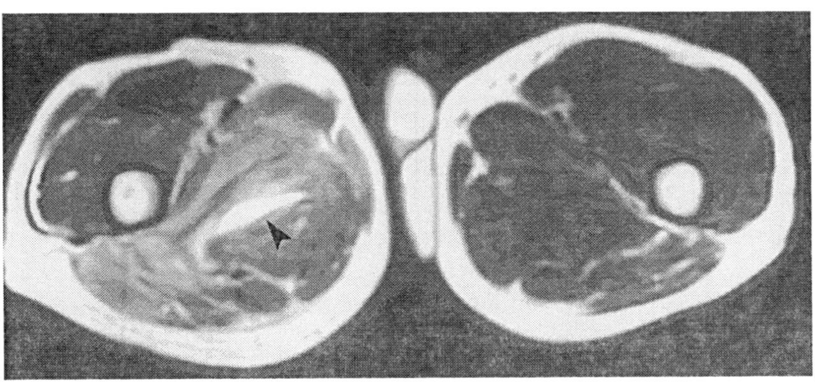

(a)

Figure 24. (Continued).

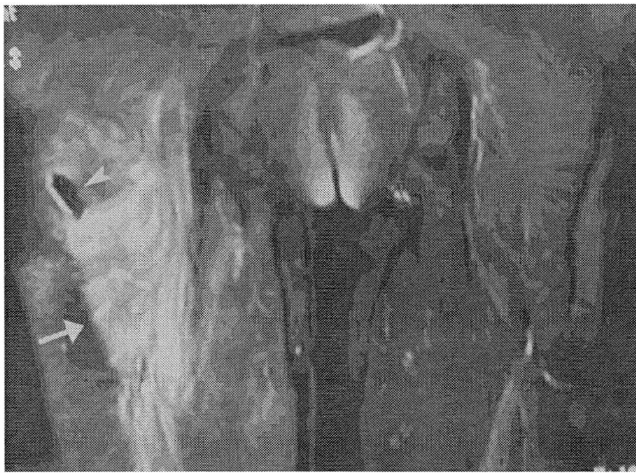

(b)

Figure 24. Skeletal muscle injury and myonecrosis. In this patient, a contaminated wound in the right thigh that occurred after a fall has led to infective myonecrosis. (a) Axial T2-weighted MR image shows the enlarged adductor and biceps femoris (muscles) with diffuse high signal intensity due to edema. Central area is seen in the adductor magnus muscle (arrowhead) consistent with a collection of fluid. (b) Coronal fat-suppressed T2-weighted MR image shows diffuse edema in the posterior compartment of the proximal thigh (arrow). Intramuscular gas with its signal void is seen (arrowhead) indicating the presence of serious infection (gas gangrene). Cultures of the infected area grew Clostridium tetani.

MRI Differential Diagnosis

In addition to the aforementioned signal intensity changes, other interesting MRI features of muscle derangement may include abnormal low signal intensity on T2-weighted images representing calcification, fibrosis, hemosiderin deposition, gas, and foreign bodies.

The presence of methemoglobin in muscle, proteinaceous material, melanin, or a gadolinium-based contrast material may account for high T1 signal intensity, in muscle. As expected, some of the conditions affecting muscle are self-limited and respond faster to conservative management, whereas others require surgical intervention and longer recovery period. Other muscle disorders however, take a more severe clinical course and are refractory to treatment, or have an ominous prognosis.

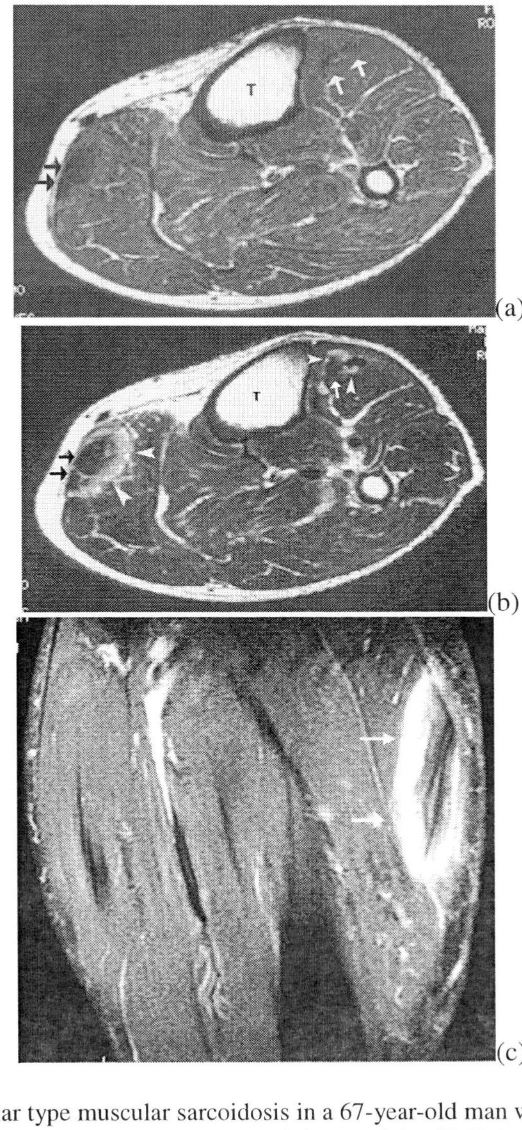

Figure 25. Nodular type muscular sarcoidosis in a 67-year-old man with painful soft tissue masses in the left thigh and leg. (a) Axial T1-weighted MR image shows low signal intensity nodules in the gastrocnemius and tibialis anterior muscles of left leg (arrows). (b) Axial T2-weighted MR image shows intramuscular calf lesions (arrows) of central low signal intensity surrounded by a thick margin of high signal intensity (arrowheads). (c) Coronal fat-suppressed T1-weighted MR image of left thigh obtained after intravenous administration of gadolinium contrast material shows large elongated lesion of central decreased signal intensity with avid rim-like enhancement in the quadriceps muscle (arrows). Biopsy disclosed noncaseating granulomas. T= tibia.

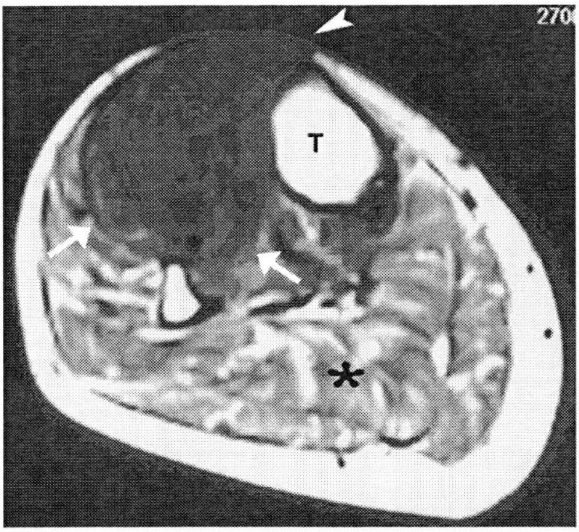

(a)

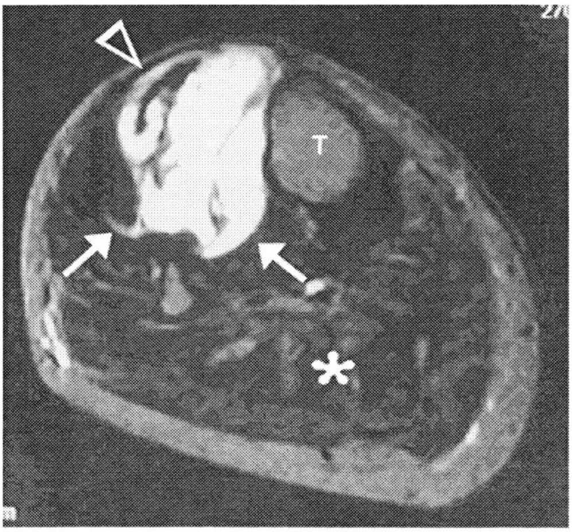

(b)

Figure 26. Leiomyosarcoma in a 78-year-old woman who presented with right leg pain,swelling, and inability to walk. (a) Axial T1-weighted MR image through calf shows large, lobular well-defined mass lesion (arrows) of predominantly low signal intensity in the tibialis anterior and tibialis posterior muscles. The mass extends to subcutaneous tissue (arrowhead). Due to diminished physical activity, muscles in the posterior compartment of the tibia show prominent fatty infiltration (asterisk). (b) Axial T2-weighted MR image with fat suppression shows intramuscular lesion of predominant high signal intensity (arrows) with peripheral necrotic region of low signal (open arrowhead). On this fat suppressed image, contrast the appearance of the low signal intensity, fat-replaced muscle in posterior tibia (asterisk) with that in part (a) where no suppression of fat was used. Biopsy of the mass lesion disclosed leiomyosarcoma of tibial muscles. T= tibia.

Conclusion

MRI plays a central role in delineating muscle anatomy and morphology, and providing characterization of muscle composition and its alterations. Although eventually biopsy may be necessary to establish diagnosis, MRI helps limit substantially the broad differential diagnosis, influencing the treatment and predicting prognosis in patients with complaints referable to muscle.

References

Fleckenstein J. L. Muscle weakness and myalgia. *MRI Clin. North Am.* 1995;3:773-790.

Powell S. T., Bracker MD. Orthopedic prespective: Muscle and tendon disease. In: Pedowitz R, Chung B, Resnick D, eds. *Magnetic resonance imaging in orthopedic sports medicine,* 1st ed. New York, NY: Springer, 2008:21-44.

Robinson G., Hine A., Richards P., Heron C. MRI abnormalities of the external rotator muscles of the hip. *Clin. Radiol.* 2005;60:401-406.

Theodorou S. J., Theodorou D. J., Resnick D. MR imaging findings of pyogenic bacterial myositis (pyomyositis) in patients with local muscle trauma: illustrative cases. *Emerg Radiol* 2007;142:89-96.

McCarthy E. F., Sundaram M. Heterotopic ossification: a review. *Skeletal Radiol* 2005;34:609-619.

Sookhoo S., MacKinnon I., Bushby K., Chinnery P., Birchall D. MRI for the demonstration of subclinical muscle involvement in muscular dystrophy. *Clinical Radiol* 2007;62:160-165.

May D., Disler D., Jones E., Balkissoon A., Manaster B. Abnormal signal intensity in skeletal muscle at MR imaging: Patterns, pearls, and pitfalls. *Radio Graphics* 2000;20:S295-315.

El-Khoury G. Y., Brandser E. A., kathol M. H., Tearse D. S., Callaghan JJ. Imaging of muscle injuries. *Skeletal. Radiol.* 1996;25:3-11.

Garcia J. MRI in inflammatory myopathies. *Skeletal Radiol* 2000;29:425-38.

Theodorou S. J., Theodorou D. J., Resnick D. Imaging findings of complications affecting the upper extremity in intravenous drug users: featured cases. *Emerg. Radiol.* 2008;15:227-239.

Elliott J., Galloway G., Jull G., Noteboom J., Centeno C., Gibbon W. Magnetic resonance imaging analysis of the upper cervical spine extensor musculature in an asymptomatic cohort: an index of fat within muscle. *Clin. Radiol.* 2005;60:355-363.

Kang C., Shin M., Kim S., Lee S., Lee C. MRI of paraspinal muscles in lumbar degenerative kyphosis patients and control patients with chronic low back pain. *Clin Radiol* 2007;62:479-486.

Kader D., Wardlaw D., Smith F. Correlation between the MRI changes in the lumbar multifidus muscles and leg pain. *Clin Radiol* 2000;55:145-149.

Moore S., Teirstein A. Musculoskeletal sarcoidosis: spectrum of appearances at MR imaging. *Radio Graphics* 2003;23:1389-1399.

Crundwell N., O'Donnell P., Saiffuddin A. Non-neoplastic conditions presenting as soft-tissue tumours. *Clinical Radiol* 2007;62:18-27.

Vilanova J. C., Woerler K., Narvaez J., Barcelo J., Martinez S., Villalon M., Miro J. Soft tissue tumors update: MR imaging features according to the WHO classification. *Eur. Radiol.* 2007;17:125-138.

In: Soft Tissue
Editors: A. J. Chavez Ruiz et al.
ISBN 978-1-62257-363-9

Chapter VI

Soft Tissue Behavior after Mandibular Syphysis Bone Graft Harvesting

***Claudio Ferreira Nóia*[*1], *Rafael Ortega Lopes*[2], *Claudinei Ferreira Nóia*[3], *and José Marcelo Vargas Pinto*[4]**

[1]Oral Diagnosis, Piracicaba Dental School, University of Campinas- Brazil
[2]Oral Diagnosis, Piracicaba Dental School, University of Campinas- Brazil
[3]School of Biomedical Sciences of Cacoal- Brazil
[4]School São Lucas- Brazil

Abstract

The use of bone graft material harvested from the mandibular symphysis to rehabilitate bone defects is considered to be a reliable procedure offering easy access and good quality bone tissue. The literature indicates the suitability of this donor area for reconstructing intra-oral defects with extensions of up to four teeth, and correcting

* E-mail: claudioferreira2004@yahoo.com.br

alveolar-palatine clefts and orbital cavity defects. Most studies involving grafts obtained from this donor region are concerned with the characteristics of the bone graft itself rather than the alterations that its removal may cause in adjacent soft tissues or precautions to be taken with them. We have sought to make a prospective assessment of neurosensory disturbances, alterations to soft tissue contours and **patients**' perceptions of the changes occurring after mandibular symphysis bone graft removal. Results show that neurosensory disturbances affect 50% of patients immediately after surgery but as the months go by that percentage reduces considerably. Soft tissue contours are altered by the procedure mainly due to the difficulty of accurately repositioning the mentalis muscles which may lead to an eversion of the lower lip compatible with labial ptosis. Patients report a perception of paresthesia in the operated region and even months afterwards that condition tends to persist However they also declare that the paresthesia does not interfere with eating, speaking or lower lip movements. Another interesting fact is that patients do not notice any alteration to the profile of the operated area. It can be concluded that the use of bone graft material removed from the mandibular symphysis region causes neurosensorial disturbances and alterations to the soft tissue contours but patients declare that those disturbances and alterations do not interfere in their daily routines.

Introduction

The use of autogenous bone grafts for re-structuring atrophied alveolar crests prior to rehabilitation with dental implant placement has become a gold standard treatment. Several studies have shown that the mandibular symphysis is a suitable donor area for such graft material offering easy access and a good quantity bone tissue of a suitable quality [1-2]. The literature also emphasizes the ready accessibility of the region, the suitable quantity and quality of the bone tissue and its ectomesenchymal origin, which ensures early vascularization and the maintenance of volume and viability during the period of its incorporation [2-4]. Currently the use of this particular donor area is indicated in cases of alveolar reconstruction involving extensions of up to four teeth, or sites involving one or two teeth that require gains in alveolar height and/or thickness. The literature also reports its use in the correction of alveolar-palatine clefts where special care is recommended to avoid any damage to permanent tooth buds[5-6]. Most studies on mandibular symphysis grafts focus on the volume and conditions of the bone graft itself rather than on procedures to take care of the soft tissues involved in the donor area or the alterations to them it may cause [7]. Thus studies are needed to accompany the alterations to soft tissues after the bone graft material has been harvested from this particular donor area. Accordingly, we have sought to make a prospective assessment of neurosensory disturbances, alterations to soft tissue contours and patients' perceptions of the changes occurring after mandibular symphysis bone harvesting.

Material and Methods

This prospective not radomized study inclued 30 patients, 22 women and 8 men, with ages ranging from 21 to 65 (average 45), treated at Piracicaba Dental Scholl by the Department of Oral and Maxillofacial Surgery, all of whom needed to undergo the harvesting of a chin bone graft to subsequent rehabilitation with implants. Were excluded in the sample patients who had undergone surgery in the chin, who had not first or second molar or the lower central incisors, and those who not agreed to participate in the study. None of the patients had any background of trauma or alterations to sensitivity in the chin region. Two surgeons conducted the operations using standard surgical techniques.

Surgical Procedure

The surgical procedure to harvest the graft involved a horizontal incision in the alveolar mucosa in the inter-canine region, 5 mm below the muco-gingival line. Subsequently an incision was made through the mentalis muscles on each side and on down to the bone. After careful raising the muco-periosteal flap at lower border of mandible and locating the mental foramina, the osteotomy was carried out using a N° 702 cross-cut fissure burr. The form of each graft block removed was determined by the reconstruction it was destined for but in every case a distance of at least 5 mm was maintained from the roots of the canine teeth, the mental nerves and the base of the mandible. The final separation and removal of the graft block was achieved using chisels. In all patients was removed 30 X 10mm corticocancellous block. Closure was carried out in two stages. The internal sutures consisted of three stitches using 3-0 suture catgut (Point Suture, Fortaleza-Brazil) and was designed to achieve precise repositioning of the mentalis muscles. A continuous suture using the same kind of catgut was used for closure of the mucosa. A microporous tape was then placed over the site to minimize edema and haematoma formation. The tape was removed 72h later.

Evaluation Method

To assess any alterations occurring in the soft tissues in the region, lateral cephalograms were taken preoperatively and postoperatively after 180 days.The cephalometric tracings were done by the same researcher on 0.07mm acetate sheet using a 0.5mm lead pencil. The analysis of soft tissue positions made use of the following parameters, based on a set of points and lines proposed by Chauschu *et al.*, (2001) [8]: Lower lip length (LLL); Exposure of the lower incisors (ELI); Vertical position of the vermilion (VPV); Vertical position of the soft tissue supramentale (VPSms); and Vertical position of the soft tissue pogonion (VPPgs) (Figure 1).

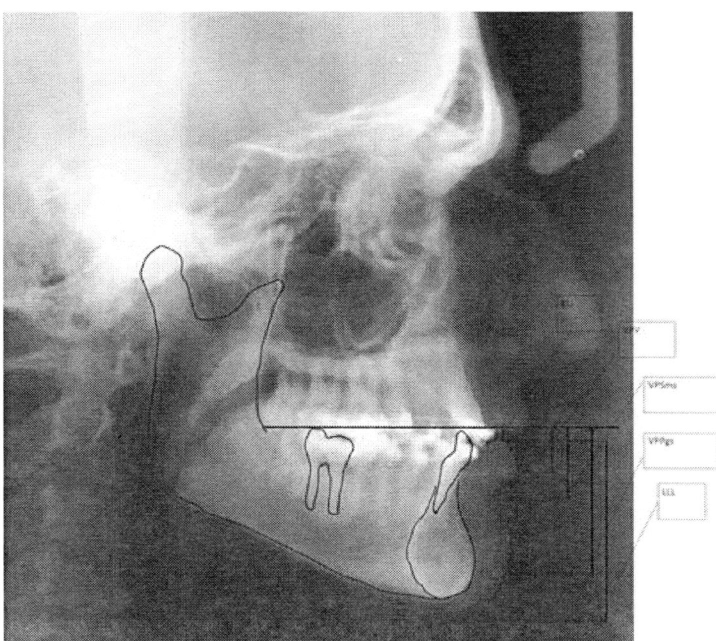

Figure 1. Reference points and lines used to evaluate changes in the vertical profile. Source: Chauschu et al., 2001 [8], adapted by the authors.

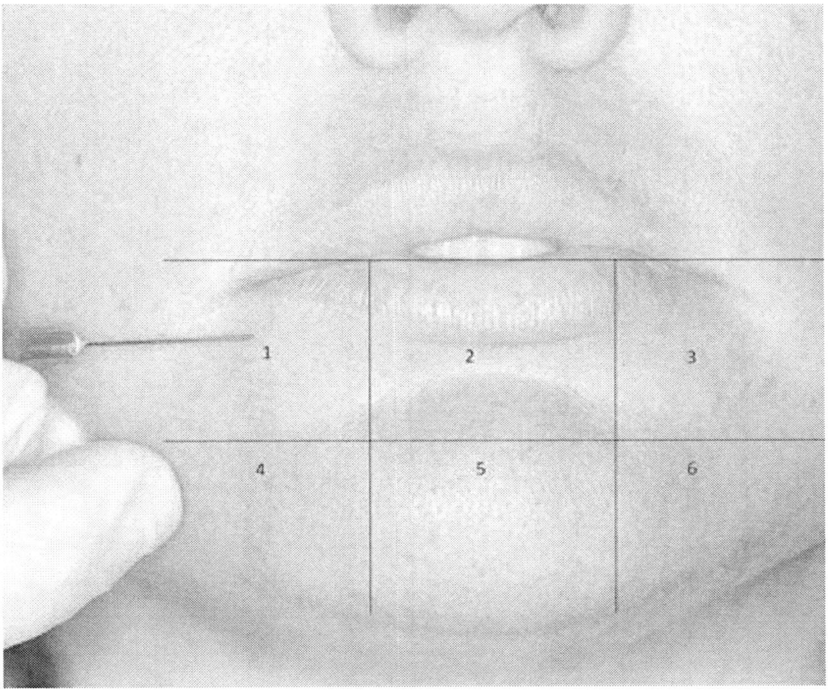

Figure 2. Pin-Prick.

One observer realized sensorial test in the pre-operatory and post-operatory period, including the first month after surgery, sixth and twelfth month. Pin-prick (PP): a needle of 25x7mm was applied on the cutaneous tissue of chin and was accepted a positive response when de patient recognized a light pain sensation (Figure 2).

Subjective evaluation of patient perception was done using Visual Analogue Scale testing –VAS. A horizontal line, 10 cm long, was the scale and patients were asked to mark an X on the line indicating their perception of the extent of alterations in the chin region after surgery. The left extremity of the line corresponded to 'no alteration' and the right to 'a lot of alteration'. The individual variables evaluated in this way were sensibility (SEN), eating (EAT), speaking (SPK) and lower lip movement (LLM). To analyze the results, the line was divided up into 2 cm-long sections corresponding to the following perceptions: section 01: no alteration; section 02: almost no alteration; section 03: a little alteration; section 04: a reasonable amount of alteration; and section 05: a lot of alteration.

Results

In the comparison between preoperative and postoperative measurements at 180 days there was a statistically significant change in the variables exposure of the lower incisors (ELI) and vertical position of the vermilion (VPV), which also had its measure increased (Table 1).

Table 1. Mean values (standard deviation) of investigated variables against time

Variable	Time	
	Preoperative	06 Months
LLL	49.46 (3.91) A	48.99 (3.90) A
VPV	10.08 (2.96) A	11.01 (2.16) B
VPSms	18.30 (3.43) A	18.62 (3.10) A
VPPgs	36.63 (3.66) A	37.03 (4.42) A
ELI	2.0 (-2; 7) A	3.5 (-3; 12) B

Different capital letters in the lines indicate statistically significant differences where $p \leq 0.05$.

The table 2 present the morbidity related to surgery and can be observed that for the first evaluation in the day 30 after surgery PP presented sensorial morbidity in 50% (15) of patients. In the sixth month evaluation, the PP test even presented 7patients (23.3%) affected by surgical morbidity. In the one year follow-up was not observed morbidity related to altered sensation, being absent all sensory complications; all patient affected return to preoperative status (Table 2).

Table 2. Number and % of patients giving negative answers in the Pin-prick

MONTH	PP
0	0(0%)
1	15(50%)
6	7(23.3%)
12	0(0%)

An analysis of the results of the subjective VAS tests shows that most patients reported a lot of alteration in sensitivity in the chin region during the first month after surgery (5), but by the six-month evaluation the alterations had diminished (4). The evaluation made 12 months after surgery shows that patients showed little loss of sensitivity (3). In regard to facial aesthetics, speech and lower lip movement, patients reported no alterations (1) at the end of the study (Table 3).

Table 3. Medians for VAS results (minimum – maximum), according to each variable and each period of evaluation

	VAS				
MONTH	SEN		EAT	SPK	LLM
0	1 (1-1) A		1 (1-1) A	1 (1-1) A	1 (1-1) A
1	5 (2-5) B		1 (1-3) A	1 (1-3) A	2 (1-4) B
6	4 (1-5) B		1 (1-3) A	1 (1-2) A	1 (1-3) A
12	3 (1-5) B		1 (1-2) A	1 (1-1) A	1 (1-2) A

Discussion

Dental implant rehabilitation seeks to restore: patient's ability to mastigate, oral comfort, facial aesthetics and speech normality, irrespective of the existence of any atrophy, disease or lesions to the stomatognathic system[9-10]. Biomaterials like autogenous, heterogenous and homogenous bone have been used to restore atrophied alveolar crests in preparation for installing dental implants. Although some controversy and discussion still persist, studies have shown that the use of autogenous bone gives the best clinical results, making the long term success of rehabilitation more reliable [1,2,6]. Most of the patients undergoing this type of grafting procedure experience some post-operational morbidity but it is transitory and considered to be acceptable [3-4].

Three types of intra-oral incision are commonly used to chin bone for graft harvesting: the sulcular, the marginal, and the alveolar mucosal [7]. This study used the alveolar mucosal incisions exclusively to avoid introducing any interference in the experiment stemming from variations in the mode of access. After graft removal the surgeons sought to reposition the mentalis muscles as accurately as possible.

The results showed alterations occurring in the vertical position of the vermillion (VPV) and the exposure of the lower incisors (ELI) with increased distances from the plane of reference as well as a drop to a lower position; a condition compatible with labial ptosis. Those findings corroborate the results obtained by Chauschu *et al.*, (2001) [8] in patients undergoing mentoplasty in which precise reattachment of the mentalis muscles was attempted but without prior identification, isolation or marking of the same.

Based on the results of this study and those of Chauschu *et al.*, (2001) [8], we can state that the bone graft harvesting from chin, cause contour changes in the soft tissue in this region, however, the changes that occurred in the soft tissues of the chin are not the direct result of harvesting the bone graft but rather of the failure to accurately reattach the mentalis muscle in its original position.

The result of research related high sensorial alteration in the first month after surgery with a 50% of sample with some grade of morbidity; this situation represent minor values when compared with the altered sensation reported by Clavero, Lundgren, (2003) [11] close to 80% of sample in the same period.

When was analyzed the sixth month after surgery, own result presented a 23.3%; Clavero, Lundgren (2003) [11] reported close to 50% of morbidity in the first year after surgery, showed a diminished of 30% from the initial evaluation; in this directions, in a 12 month period, Joshi (2004) [12] observed 33% of sensorial alteration; in our research was not observed morbidity in a 12 month period. We believe that this differences can be associated to surgical technique, amount of bone removed, instruments used in the osteotomy (quality of the drills and refrigeration, for example) and depth of osteotomy.

This study the subjective evaluation using VAS technique showed that facial aesthetics, eating, speech and lower lip movements were practically unaffected by the harvesting of chin bone grafts. Sensitivity in the region, however, showed considerable alteration, but, as the postoperative period progressed, the situation steadily improved and by the end of the study most of the patients reported relatively little alteration. Similar results have been reported by Raghoebar *et al.*, (2001) [13], Mazzonetto *et al.*, (2004) [14], Booij et al., (2005) [15], and Weibull *et al.*, (2009) [3], all of whom assessed subjective impressions of patients undergoing this type of bone graft surgery and also observed that most patients reported alterations in sensitivity. The authors noted that patient's daily routines were unaffected, and that most of them had a positive opinion of the surgery and would readily submit to it again, should it prove necessary.

Conclusion

It can be concluded that the use of bone graft material removed from the mandibular symphysis region causes neurosensorial disturbances and alterations to the soft tissue contours but patients declare that those disturbances and alterations do not interfere in their daily routines.

References

[1] Triplett RG, Schow SR. Autologous bone grafts and endosseous implants: complementary techniques. *J Oral Maxillofac Surg*. 1996; 54:486-94.

[2] Misch CE. Comparison of intraoral donor sites for onlay grafting prior to implant placement. *Int J Oral Maxillofac Implants*. 1997;12:767-76.

[3] Weibull L, Widmark G, Ivanoff C, Borg E, Rasmusson L. Morbidity after chin bone harvesting – A retrospective long-term follow-up study. *Clin Impl Dent Relat Res*. 2009; 11: 149-157.

[4] Von Arx T, Hafliger J, Chappuis V. Neurosensory disturbances following bone harvesting in the symphysis: a prospective clinical study. *Clin Oral Impl Res*. 2005;12:432-9.

[5] Dik EA, Ruiter AP, Van der Bilt A, Koole R. Effect on the contour of bone and soft tissue one year after harvesting chin bone for alveolar cleft repair. *Int J Oral Maxillofac Surg*. 2010; 39: 962-967.

[6] Branemark PI, Lindstrom J, Hallén O, Breine U, Jeppson P-H, Ohman A. Reconstruction of the defective mandible. *Scand J Plast Reconstr Surg*. 1975;9:116-28.

[7] Gapski R, Wang HL, Misch CE. Management of incision design in symphysis graft procedures: A review of the literature. *J Oral Implantology*. 2001;27:134-42.

[8] Chaushu G, Blinder D, Taicher S, Chaushu S. The effect of precise reattachment of the mentalis muscle on the soft tissue response to genioplasty. *J Oral Maxillofac Surg* 2001; 59: 510-516.

[9] Rodríguez-Chessa JG. Tratamento de maxilas atróficas por meio de fixações zigomáticas. *Análise retrospectiva de 03 anos [Tese]. Piracicaba: UNICAMP/FOP;* 2009.

[10] Nóia CF. Avaliação radiográfica prospectiva de alterações estéticas em pacientes submetidos à remoção de enxerto de mento [Dissertação]. *Piracicaba: UNICAMP/FOP*; 2011.

[11] Clavero J and Lundgren S. Ramus or chin grafts for maxillary sinus inlay and local onlay augmentation: comparison of donor site morbidity and complications. *Clin Implant Dent Res* 2003; 5: 154-60.

[12] Joshi A. An investigation of post-operative morbidity following chin graft surgery. *Br Dent J.* 2004;196:215-8.

[13] Raghoebar GM, Louwerse C, Kalk WWI and Vissink A. Morbidity of chin bone harvesting. *Clin Oral Implants Res.* 2001; 12: 503-7.

[14] Mazzonetto R, Bozza PA, Luvisotto SG. Análise subjetiva de pacientes submetidos à cirurgia de enxerto ósseo Autógeno de mento. *Rev Assoc Paul Cir Dent.* 2004;58:263-8.

[15] Booij A, Raghoebar GM, Jansma J, Kalk WWI, Vissink A. Morbidity of chin bone transplants used for reconstructing alveolar defects in cleft patients. *Cleft Palate-Caniofac J.* 2005; 42: 533-538.

Index

A

B

C

D

E

F

G

H

I

J

K

L

M

N

O

P

Q

R

S

T